Communication and Swallowing Changes in Healthy Aging Adults

Angela N. Burda, PhD, CCC-SLP
Associate Professor
Department of Communication Sciences and Disorders
University of Northern Iowa
Cedar Falls, Iowa

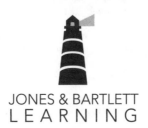
JONES & BARTLETT
LEARNING

World Headquarters
Jones & Bartlett Learning
40 Tall Pine Drive
Sudbury, MA 01776
978-443-5000
info@jblearning.com
www.jblearning.com

Jones & Bartlett Learning
Canada
6339 Ormindale Way
Mississauga, Ontario L5V 1J2
Canada

Jones & Bartlett Learning
International
Barb House, Barb Mews
London W6 7PA
United Kingdom

Jones & Bartlett Learning books and products are available through most bookstores and online booksellers. To contact Jones & Bartlett Learning directly, call 800-832-0034, fax 978-443-8000, or visit our website www.jblearning.com.

Substantial discounts on bulk quantities of Jones & Bartlett Learning publications are available to corporations, professional associations, and other qualified organizations. For details and specific discount information, contact the special sales department at Jones & Bartlett Learning via the above contact information or send an email to specialsales@jblearning.com.

Production Credits
Publisher: David Cella
Associate Editor: Maro Gartside
Editorial Assistant: Teresa Reilly
Production Manager: Julie Champagne Bolduc
Associate Production Editor: Jessica Steele Newfell
Marketing Manager: Grace Richards
Manufacturing and Inventory Control Supervisor: Amy Bacus
Composition: Glyph International
Cover Design: Kristin E. Parker
Cover and Chapter-Opening Image: © Kervie Mata/Dreamstime.com
Printing and Binding: Malloy, Inc.
Cover Printing: Malloy, Inc.

Library of Congress Cataloging-in-Publication Data
Communication and swallowing changes in healthy aging adults / edited by Angela N. Burda.
    p. ; cm.
  Includes bibliographical references and index.
  ISBN 978-0-7637-7656-5 (pbk. : alk. paper) 1. Senses and sensation in old age. 2. Deglutition.
3. Esophagus—Aging. 4. Communicative disorders in old age. 5. Deglutition disorders—Age factors. I. Burda, Angela N.
  [DNLM: 1. Aging—physiology. 2. Aged. 3. Communication. 4. Comprehension—physiology. 5. Deglutition—physiology. 6. Geriatric Assessment. WT 104 C7336 2011]
  QP435.C66 2011
  612.8—dc22
                                                                    2010002617

6048

Printed in the United States of America
14 13 12 11 10   10 9 8 7 6 5 4 3 2 1

Contents

Preface

According to the American Speech-Language-Hearing Association, approximately 39,000 speech-language pathologists (SLPs) work in healthcare facilities, with 6000 currently working in long-term care facilities. It is likely that many of the patients these SLPs see are elderly adults. Fortunately, our discipline has a significant amount of literature available on the kinds of cognitive-linguistic, motor speech, and swallowing impairments that older adults may have as a result of strokes, head injuries, and disease processes such as Alzheimer's disease or Parkinson's disease. What our field is lacking, however, is normative information as to what SLPs can expect from healthy older adults. Lack of such data does not allow SLPs to fully compare what would be considered normal for their elderly patients versus what is considered pathological. Without knowing what would be considered within the spectrum of normal, SLPs may not address therapy as effectively as possible. They may overestimate or underestimate what aging adults are capable of doing. Yet, medically based SLPs must evaluate patients and typically make treatment decisions quickly. Thus, this book was written to serve as a resource for SLPs and assist them in determining their course of evaluation and treatment of their elderly patients. This book was also developed to provide SLP students with useful information when learning about the aging population. In addition, several of the chapters contain original data not published elsewhere. The final chapter discusses the communication abilities and health of aging adults in a much broader fashion using the World Health Organization's *International Classification of Functioning, Disability, and Health*, an increasingly important perspective of which to be knowledgeable. I hope that readers of all levels, whether students or practicing professionals, find this text helpful.

Acknowledgments

I have been extremely fortunate to have had many wonderful individuals involved in this project. Although it has been a marathon, it has also been an experience in which I have learned a great deal. First and foremost, I certainly appreciate the willingness of Jones & Bartlett Learning to give me this opportunity. Dave Cella, Publisher, and Maro Gartside, Associate Editor, at Jones & Bartlett Learning have been incredibly helpful throughout the entire process. I also appreciate the useful feedback provided by the reviewers. I am grateful to be a 2007 and 2008 recipient of the University of Northern Iowa's Adele Whitenack Davis Faculty Research in Gerontology Award. These funding opportunities allowed me to conduct research pertinent to this book, which I have included in Chapters 2 through 6. Special thanks to the contributing authors: Todd Bohnenkamp, Jill Champley, Julia Edgar, Carlin Hageman, and Travis Threats. They are friends and colleagues who kindly agreed to share their expertise. A huge "thank you" goes out to my graduate assistants and students who worked long and hard to help me out on this endeavor: Andrea Bakeris, Alison Corbett, Ashley Cox, Holly Drury, Stephanie Jones, Beth Kluesner, Laci Kuker, Bekah Rickels, Leslie Spalding, Janet Thomas, and Laura Wright. Special thanks to the (self-proclaimed) "Cool Kids" in my spring 2008 Acquired Cognitive Disorders seminar for providing their feedback on Chapter 2: Jamie Flatness, Laci Kuker, Brandi Lawrance, Alisha Sanchez, Jenny Scharn, Sara Smith, Tally Stowell, and Janet Thomas. Special thanks also goes out to the students in my fall 2009 Speech-Language Pathology (SLP) Issues in Aging and Accent seminar for their help with the discussion questions: Andrea Bakeris, Ashley Cox, LeAnn Gaughan, Julie Hennessy, Meghan Kelly, Jennifer Kemps, Beth Kluesner, Lindsey Schoening, Leslie Spalding, and Jacayla Vittetoe.

My parents, Dick and Jan, my sister Susan, her boyfriend Charlie, and my Grandma Jacky have always been a great source of support. I am lucky to have such a great family. Thanks, Deb for everything, especially all of your kind words. Kim, you and I lead parallel lives, and I always appreciate your encouragement. To my husband, Jim, words cannot express how much your kindness, love, and support every day mean to me. Thanks for being my number-one fan.

About the Author

Angela N. Burda is an Associate Professor in the Department of Communication Sciences and Disorders at the University of Northern Iowa (UNI). Dr. Burda obtained her BA and MA degrees from the University of Minnesota–Duluth and her PhD from Wichita State University. She has been at UNI since 2000 and teaches courses in acquired neurogenic disorders, normal aging, and accent modification. Her primary areas of research include investigating cognitive-linguistic performance in healthy middle-aged and older adults and the understanding of accented speech by aging adults. She has published several articles and presented her research regionally, nationally, and internationally. Prior to working in academe, Dr. Burda worked as a speech-language pathologist in rehabilitation hospitals and long-term care facilities in St. Paul, Minnesota, and Wichita, Kansas.

Contributing Authors

Todd A. Bohnenkamp, PhD, CCC-SLP
Assistant Professor
Department of Communication Sciences and Disorders
University of Northern Iowa
Cedar Falls, Iowa

Jill L. Champley, PhD, CCC-SLP
Speech-Language Pathologist
VA Nebraska–Western Iowa Health Care System
Omaha, Nebraska

Julia D. Edgar, PhD, CCC-SLP
Research Scientist
Department of Otolaryngology–Research
Washington University School of Medicine
St. Louis, Missouri

Carlin F. Hageman, PhD, CCC-SLP
Professor and Department Head
Department of Communication Sciences and Disorders
University of Northern Iowa
Cedar Falls, Iowa

Travis T. Threats, PhD, CCC-SLP
Professor and Chair
Department of Communication Sciences and Disorders
St. Louis University
St. Louis, Missouri

Chapter 1

Introduction and Theoretical Perspectives

Angela N. Burda, PhD, CCC-SLP

Introduction

With the rapid aging of populations in the United States and in many countries around the world, there is a need for speech-language pathologists (SLPs) to know what is considered normal for older adults in terms of cognitive-linguistic, motor speech, voice, and swallowing abilities. This need coincides with the continuing quest for evidence-based practice (EBP) in the field of speech-language pathology (Reilly, Douglas, & Oates, 2004). Having normative data will help SLPs meet the EBP guidelines described in a position statement developed by the American Speech-Language-Hearing Association (ASHA, 2005). The position paper in part states that professionals must recognize the needs and abilities "of individuals and families to whom they provide clinical services, and integrate those factors along with best current research evidence and their clinical expertise in making clinical decisions." In addition, SLPs need to "acquire and maintain the knowledge and skills that are necessary to provide high quality professional services, including knowledge and skills related to evidence-based practice" (ASHA, 2005, p.1).

Thus, the information presented in this book is meant to help SLPs make decisions about assessment and treatment protocols for their elderly patients. Professionals must also learn how to view the health of aging adults in a much broader fashion using the World Health Organization's (WHO) *International Classification of Functioning, Disability, and Health*.

Chapters 2 through 8 of this book are organized in a similar format: for each topic, older adults' general abilities are presented, followed by a description of factors that negatively affect those abilities, and signs of problems that warrant referrals to professionals. Helpful strategies for dealing with these problems are then discussed. The final chapter discusses the WHO framework and its application to the aging population. Each chapter concludes with a list of "Quick Facts" summarizing key points, as well as a set of discussion questions. A Glossary of potentially unfamiliar terms is included, as well as an Appendix that lists tests SLPs can use to evaluate their adult clients. Pros and cons of each test are presented. This current chapter gives operational definitions pertinent to the book, and it presents theoretical perspectives regarding age-related changes affecting cognition and language. As with the other chapters in this book, "Quick Facts" and discussion questions are included at the end.

Operational Definitions: Healthy and Older

What is healthy? At what age is one considered *older*? Although both terms seem to be easily understood, in actuality, finding adequate definitions is somewhat challenging. Many research studies include healthy older adults as participants, but very few actually state what they mean by *healthy*. Similar to what other authors do (Cohn, Dustman, & Bradford, 1984; Collie, Shafiq-Antonacci, Maruff, Tyler, & Currie, 1999; Meijer, De Groot, Van Boxtel, Van Gerven, & Jolles, 2006), in this book we use *healthy* to refer to the lack of any kind of neurological disease or disorder, such as stroke, dementia, or progressive diseases such as Alzheimer's disease and multiple sclerosis, that would presumably interfere with the abilities discussed (e.g., auditory comprehension, swallowing). However, some investigators use additional criteria when classifying their healthy older adult groups. For example, Collie and colleagues (1999) stated that participants in their study could not have epilepsy, diabetes, thyroid disease, major depression/anxiety, or other psychiatric illness. Carlson, Fried, Xue, Bandeen-Roche, Zeger, and Brandt (1999) included aging adults who were physically high functioning and cognitively intact in their study. The absence of neurological damage is key because its presence, even if seemingly resolved, as in the case of transient ischemic attacks (Shankle & Amen, 2005), can easily affect the abilities described in this book. In some cases, researchers use the terms normal or neurologically intact synonymously with the word healthy (Peel, Bartlett, & McClure, 2004).

Defining aging or older is not any easier. Qualifications seem to span the gamut. Many people are quite surprised when they receive their first complimentary issue of the AARP (American Association of Retired Persons) magazine at the age of 50. Many 70-year-olds feel as energetic and healthy as ever and believe the number of birthdays they have celebrated does not necessarily reflect the vitality they feel (Stephens, 1991). Research articles are not any more helpful. Some studies classify older adults as being in their 50s and older (Constantinidou & Baker, 2002; De Beni, Palladino, Borella, & Lo Presti, 2003; Federmeier, Van Petten, Schwartz, & Kutas, 2003), while other investigations consider individuals "older" at age 65 and above (Gordon-Salant & Fitzgibbons, 1999; Little, Prentice, Darrow, & Wingfield, 2005; Pichora-Fuller, Schneider, & Daneman, 1995). Many studies do not specify a maximum age, allowing adults in their 80s and 90s to participate (Burda, 2007, 2008; De Beni et al., 2003; Kemper, 1986; Parkin & Java, 1999). The classifications of young-old, middle-old, and old-old can also be used and typically begin at age 65 and progress upward (Burda, 2007, 2008; Schmitt, 1983). For this book, aging and older in general refer to individuals who are age 65 and older. However, it should be noted that in some cases, adults in their 50s may also fall into this category because a valuable research study has included them as part of the older adult participant group (e.g., De Beni et al., 2003; Federmeier et al., 2003).

Although age-related changes can be evident in the various abilities discussed in this book, possessing these skills to an adequate degree factors heavily into older adults' overall health and well-being (Shadden & Toner, 1997; Worrall & Hickson, 2003). Older adults who are in generally good health tend to feel younger than their chronological age (Gana, Alaphilippe, & Bailly, 2004). Conversely, aging adults in poor health tend to feel quite the opposite (Logan, Ward, & Spitze, 1992; Nakamura, Moritani, & Kanetaka, 1989). The majority of changes noted in the book happen gradually (Buckner, Head, & Lustig, 2006), differing significantly from the rapid neurological changes of early childhood. Although there are reports stating that physical and mental abilities peak in the 20s (Hutchinson, 2008; Skirbekk, 2003), plenty in the literature details the rewards of aging, such as mastering professional skills and hobbies (Abraham & Hansson, 1995; Ericsson & Kintsch, 1995), growing confidence (MacKinlay, 2006), and enjoying rich relationships with loved ones, friends, and colleagues (Adams & Blieszner, 1995). Thus, while the upcoming chapters often describe declines in abilities (Rabbitt & Anderson, 2006), these changes should not necessarily nor absolutely be viewed as losses. Yes, it is irritating to forget someone's name or to not be able to recall a piece of information as quickly as one wants, but such changes do not mean that older individuals have a poorer quality of life. Many would indeed argue otherwise.

Theoretical Perspectives

Many age-related cognitive theories have been developed and evaluated over the years. Despite the significant amount of literature available, no clear-cut theory has emerged to explain the underlying cognitive-linguistic changes that occur during aging. However, it may be impossible for one theory to account for the various changes that can affect so many different areas (Thornton & Light, 2006). Although this book rather tidily discusses specific abilities of older adults (e.g., auditory comprehension, writing), the reality is that these abilities often overlap. For example, intact attention and memory are needed so that individuals can comprehend questions asked of them and then formulate appropriate responses. Not only do abilities overlap, so can the theories presented, because they tend to encompass broad frameworks (Light, 1991; MacKay & James, 2001; Thornton & Light, 2006). Although these theories generally address underlying cognitive changes, such changes obviously will in turn affect comprehension and expression abilities. As Thornton and Light (2006) note, cognitive aging theories are generally applied in order to interpret normal age-related language changes. The rest of this chapter is meant to serve as a tutorial by presenting some of the most widely studied age-related cognitive theories. Although studies are discussed that support each of the theories, there are just as many investigations published that refute or question them. The following theories are presented: inhibition deficit, transmission deficit, cognitive slowing, and reduced resources, including reduced working memory abilities. A view that hypothesizes that neurobiological changes cause age-related cognitive declines is also discussed.

Inhibition Deficit

The inhibition deficit hypothesis posits that aging weakens inhibitory processes, making it more difficult for older adults to suppress irrelevant information compared with young adults (Hasher & Zacks, 1988; Zacks & Hasher, 1997). For example, older adults have greater difficulty ignoring a distracting word that is printed in a different typeface (Connelly, Hasher, & Zacks, 1991; Zacks & Hasher, 1997). Such distractions slow aging adults' reading and negatively impact their comprehension and memory of the text (Connelly et al., 1991; Zacks & Hasher, 1997). The presence of distracting speech can also adversely affect older adults' recall abilities. Tun, O'Kane, and Wingfield (2002) had younger and older adults listen to word lists presented in English while ignoring competing speech spoken in English (considered meaningful) or Dutch (considered meaningless). They found that older adults had greater difficulty compared with the younger adults in ignoring the competing speech and had poorer recall of the target words. They also had the poorest performance when the competing speech was presented in English.

Other investigations on the inhibition deficit hypothesis involve word-retrieval or word-recognition tasks. To understand these studies, a few terms first need to be defined. Neighborhood refers to a group of words that differ from the target word by changing only one phoneme (Thornton & Light, 2006). An example of a neighborhood for the word dog would be dig, bog, log, and dock. The total number of neighbors that a target word has is referred to as neighborhood density (Thornton & Light, 2006). A word like cat resides in a high-density neighborhood because so many phonetically similar variations of the word can be obtained, such as mat, that, and cab, while a word like wolf resides in a low-density neighborhood because it has far fewer phonetically similar possibilities (J. D. Anderson, 2007). Neighborhood frequency indicates how often those neighbors are used (Thornton & Light, 2006).

Researchers have reported that older adults have greater difficulty than younger adults in identifying low-frequency words in high-density neighborhoods (Sommers, 1996; Sommers & Danielson, 1999). Examples of such words include dot, pet, and cake (Munson, 2007). However, context can help older adults perform generally as accurately as young adults, specifically when these words are used in highly constrained sentences (e.g., "The accident gave me a scare" versus "Ms. Smith considered the scare"). Sommers and Danielson (1999) theorized that aging adults' challenges with identifying low-frequency, high-density words shows their difficulty in inhibiting higher-frequency, phonologically similar words, leading to processing difficulties. In addition to neighborhood density, other investigators have reported that word length and word frequency can affect older adults' naming abilities (Spieler & Balota, 2000; Whiting et al., 2003). For example, older adults can have greater difficulty accessing the name of lower-frequency words (Spieler & Balota, 2000). Examples of low-frequency words are brood and wool (Whiting et al., 2003). Thus, the basis of the inhibition deficit hypothesis is that the inability to ignore the presence of distracting and/or competing information or thoughts makes it more difficult for older adults to accurately process and carry out various tasks.

Transmission Deficit

The transmission deficit account proposes that age-related cognitive changes occur because memory connections are weakened, leading to poorer activation of the target information (Burke, MacKay, Worthley, & Wade, 1991; James & Burke, 2000; MacKay & James, 2004). Semantic knowledge is organized into networks of nodes (i.e., concepts) connected via associated pathways (J. A. Anderson, 1983; Light, 1991). Findings from studies of tip-of-the-tongue experiences (TOTs) are often used to support this theory. TOTs were first defined by Brown and McNeill (1966) in their seminal study as the inability to recall a known word at a time when "recall is felt imminent" (p. 325). Similarly, Schwartz (2002) more recently noted, "A TOT is a strong feeling that a target word, although currently unrecallable, is known and will be recalled" (p. 5).

TOTs increase with age and most frequently when recalling proper names and infrequently used words (Burke et al., 1991; Mortensen, Meyer, & Humphreys, 2006; Schwartz, 2002). It is believed that common names have more interconnections in memory and are more easily retrieved than proper names that are not as semantically interconnected and, therefore, have weaker connections (Thornton & Light, 2006). For example, James (2004) recently reported that older adults had more TOTs for a word when it was presented as a proper name (e.g., Mr. Farmer) versus when it was presented as an occupation (e.g., farmer), highlighting that semantic interconnections appeared to be stronger for common names than proper names. Maylor (1997) notes that the names of more common objects may also be easier for aging adults to retrieve because there may be more than one acceptable name for the item (e.g., cup, mug), whereas this is not usually the case for proper names. The concepts of neighborhood density and neighborhood frequency are also found in the literature regarding this particular theory. For example, older adults have more TOTs for words with low neighborhood frequencies, such as lull, joke, and palm (Vitevitch & Sommers, 2003). Such findings are interpreted to mean that words with high neighborhood frequencies have stronger memory interconnections, receive increased activation from their neighbors, and are more easily recalled (Thornton & Light, 2006).

Schwartz (2002) notes that when applying the transmission deficit theory to TOTs, it is assumed that a semantic level of representation and a phonological level of representation exist. For example, a person provided the definition "a device for protecting from rain or sun" (p. 52) may be able to evoke the meaning of the object and perhaps even visualize that object, but may not be able to access the phonological representation of the actual word umbrella (Schwartz, 2002). Low-frequency words (e.g., kiosk, sump) and words that have not been recently retrieved tend to lead to more TOTs than high-frequency words (e.g., house, girl) and words that have been accessed recently (Gollan & Silverberg, 2001; Schwartz, 2002).

Although aging weakens the link between semantic and phonological representations, leading to more TOTs in older adults (Mortensen et al., 2006; Rastle & Burke, 1996; Schwartz, 2002), the connections between these two levels improve with greater use (Schwartz, 2002). Hence, it would be reasonable to assume that strengthening such connections would reduce TOTs in aging adults. For example, White and Abrams (1999) and James and Burke (2000) found that when older adults could not retrieve a target word when given a definition (e.g., "What word means to formally renounce a throne?" Answer: "Abdicate"), they resolved more TOTs when given a prime that shared some phonological component of one of the syllables of the target word (e.g., *ab*stract, *in*digent, lo*cate*). White and Abrams (1999) reported that aging adults did best specifically when given a phonologically related prime for the first syllable (e.g., *ab*stract). Such improved performance indicates that the presentation of these additional words did not lead to difficulty suppressing irrelevant or competing information but instead demonstrated that with the appropriate assistance, weak connections were strengthened and ultimately led to improved retrieval (James & Burke, 2000; Thornton & Light, 2006).

Cognitive Slowing

Cognitive slowing has been theorized to be an underlying reason for age-related cognitive declines (Salthouse, 1996). Such slowing encompasses slower processing speed, reduced attentional abilities, and reduced working memory abilities. Although some believe that reduced attention and working memory can stand separately as theoretical underpinnings for cognitive changes in older adults (see next section), others view these reductions in a broader perspective (Salthouse, 1996). As Light (1991) notes, the relationship among these three components is complex and difficult to differentiate. Although no single reason for generalized slowing has been determined, it has been hypothesized to result from greater noise in the nervous system (Salthouse & Lichty, 1985), broken or reduced neural connections (Cerella, 1990), or an increased proportion in the loss of information at each step of processing (Salthouse, 1985).

Generalized slowing has been associated with older adults' challenges in language comprehension and recollection (Kemper, 2006). For example, aging adults have greater difficulty recalling speech segments that are presented at a faster rate but do well when speech segments are presented at a normal speaking rate (Wingfield, Tun, & Rosen, 1995). In studies in which individuals can control how fast speech segments are presented as well as the length of the segments they must listen to, older adults tend to choose slower speech rates and smaller segments (Wingfield & Ducharme, 1999; Wingfield, Lahar, & Stine, 1989). Slowing can also occur when reading. Older adults who demonstrate good recall of information spend more time reading an entire passage and syntactically complex sentences, whereas young adults spend more time reading infrequent words and new concepts presented for the first time in the text (Stine-Morrow, Loveless, & Soederberg, 1996). Investigations measuring the rate of rehearsal during memory tasks (Salthouse, 1990) and the rate of visual scanning on memory searches

(Cerella, 1985) report that aging adults have slower responses. Interestingly, Myerson, Hale, Wagstaff, Poon, and Smith (1990) point out that allowing older adults more time to complete a target task does not lead to improved performance.

Reduced Resources, Reduced Working Memory

The belief behind this theory is that older adults have fewer processing resources available to them than younger adults, causing age-linked deficits when these resources are exceeded (MacKay & James, 2001; Light, 1991). For example, listeners must rapidly identify and process individual speech sounds and words, then integrate other incoming words and sentences with what was previously spoken or stored (Pichora-Fuller et al., 1995; Thornton & Light, 2006). Auditory processing can become more effortful for aging adults if they have any degree of hearing loss, or if other variables are present, such as background noise or if more than one person is speaking simultaneously (Humes, 1996; Schneider, Daneman, Murphy, & Kwong-See, 2000; van Rooij & Plomp, 1990). In such cases, older adults must reallocate their cognitive resources and use other means to process incoming information, such as top-down processing. Top-down processing means that listeners have to rely on their own knowledge of the world and the context of the message to help them make sense out of what they are hearing. The challenge is that when aging adults become more dependent upon top-down processing, they have fewer resources available to focus on what the speaker is saying, possibly missing valuable information. In contrast, reading studies have shown that while older adults may read more slowly at the beginning of a passage, possibly to establish general comprehension of the text, they read more quickly as they proceed through the passage (Stine-Morrow, Gagne, Morrow, & DeWall, 2004; Stine-Morrow, Miller, & Leno, 2001), possibly freeing up cognitive resources to focus on new or unfamiliar information.

As previously noted, some authors do not separate reduced resources (e.g., attention) and reduced working memory from cognitive slowing (Salthouse, 1988a, 1988b). Others believe that a reduction in working memory is the reason for age-related cognitive difficulties (Caplan & Waters, 1999; Waters & Caplan, 1996, 2001, 2005). Working memory requires individuals to manipulate, store, and transform pieces of information (Baddeley, 2003), such as when mentally calculating the tip to leave at a restaurant. Older adults have declines in their working memory (Connor, 2001; Craik, 2000), and such declines have been hypothesized to occur as the result of less storage capacities (Zacks & Hasher, 1988), reduced efficiency in carrying out the needed operations (Stine & Wingfield, 1987), and mental slowing (Salthouse, 1990). Waters and Caplan (2001, 2005) further speculate that a general working memory decline may be too broad to explain age-related language declines, and that more specific interpretations are needed (e.g., a theory addressing reduced working memory negatively affecting sentence comprehension).

Researchers have found that when working-memory tasks are sufficiently difficult, such as repeating complex sentences or completing backward digit-span tasks (i.e., repeating a string of numbers in reverse order), younger adults perform better than older individuals (Kemper, 1986; Light, 1991; Salthouse, Kausler, & Saults, 1988). Age-related changes in working memory can also lead to less grammatically and syntactically complex language (Kemper, Herman, & Lian, 2003; Kemper & Sumner, 2001). Kemper, Marquis, and Thompson (2001) elicited autobiographical narratives over the course of 7–17 years from adults who were ages 65–75 at the first assessment and ages 79–83 at the final assessment. Sample questions included "Describe the persons who most influenced your life" and "Describe an unexpected event that happened to you." Measures were taken on propositional density and grammatical complexity. Propositional density refers to how much information is conveyed relative to the number of words spoken (Kemper & Sumner, 2001). The most significant declines in grammatical complexity and propositional density (i.e., individuals use more words to convey a message) occurred between the ages of 74 and 78 with more gradual declines before and after that interval. However, there was considerable individual variation in older adults' initial levels of grammatical complexity and propositional density as well as in their levels of decline. In addition, older adults' discourse is often rated as more interesting and informative than that of younger adults (James, Burke, Austin, & Hulme, 1998). Aging adults are also able to modify their speech when talking to children and persons with cognitive impairments (Adams, Smith, Pasupathi, & Vitolo, 2002; Kemper, Anagnopoulos, Lyons, & Heberlein, 1994), suggesting that their working memory abilities are adequate for keeping in mind the content of what they want to say while they alter their speech to accommodate listeners' comprehension levels.

Neurobiological Changes

Proponents of this theory report that neurobiological changes are at the root of normal age-related cognitive declines, and this pattern of decline in healthy aging adults (e.g., difficulties in attention, working memory, executive functions) is quite similar to the neuropsychological profile of persons who have damage to the prefrontal cortex (Braver et al., 2001; Moscovitch & Wincour, 1995; Perfect, 1997; Salat, Kaye, & Janowsky, 1999; West, 1996). It is well documented that older adults exhibit a reduction in brain volume and ventricular enlargement compared with younger adults (Buckner et al., 2006; Davis & Wright, 1977). Although brain volume reduction generally begins appearing after the age of 60, the area affected the earliest and to the largest degree is in the frontal cortex (Haug & Eggers, 1991; Salat et al., 1999). For example, healthy older adults do not completely activate areas in the frontal cortex to the same level that young adults do (Logan, Sanders, Snyder, Morris, & Buckner, 2002; Nyberg et al., 2003) when memorizing faces (Grady et al., 1995) or purposefully committing information to memory (Buckner, Kelley, & Petersen, 1999; Fletcher & Henson, 2001).

These cognitive declines in older adults are also thought to be associated with age-related reductions in the dopamine neurochemical system (Arnsten, Cai, Steere, & Goldman-Rakic, 1995; Li & Lindenberger, 1999; Li, Lindenberger, & Frensch, 2000; Li, Lindenberger, & Sikstrom, 2001), which Braver and colleagues (2001) believe regulates the prefrontal cortex. Based on studies that report dopamine reductions in aging, it would be reasonable to assume that increasing the level of dopamine through the use of pharmacological agents (e.g., Levodopa) would possibly stop or reverse such cognitive declines. In reality, aging adults have fewer dopamine receptors in the prefrontal cortex (Suhara et al., 1991), which might not allow such medications to work fully (Braver et al., 2001). Others report that age-related cognitive declines result from deficits involving not only the frontal cortex and basal ganglia, but also the hippocampus and associated structures in the medial temporal lobe (Buckner et al., 2006).

Conclusion

In conclusion, the aging process can affect a multitude of abilities assessed by SLPs. Although the literature reports a great deal of information on these abilities in older adults, defining *healthy* and *older* can be somewhat ambiguous. In addition, many theories have been hypothesized in order to account for age-related changes in cognition and language. As of yet, however, no single theory has emerged to explain the multitude of changes that aging adults demonstrate. Despite the declines that are reported in the upcoming chapters, many older adults enjoy vital and fulfilling lives.

Quick Facts

- General Information:
  - SLPs need to know what is considered normal for older adults' cognitive-linguistic, motor speech, voice, and swallowing abilities
  - SLPs must learn to view the health of aging adults in a broader sense using the WHO's *International Classification of Functioning, Disability, and Health*

- These needs coincide with the continuing quest for EBP in the field of speech-language pathology
- Operational Definitions for This Book:
  - *Healthy* refers to the lack of any kind of neurological disease or disorder (e.g., stroke, dementia) that would interfere with the abilities discussed in this book
  - The terms *normal* and *neurologically intact* may be used synonymously with the word *healthy*
  - In research studies, *aging* and *older* generally refer to individuals aged 65 and older, but some studies have included adults in their 50s
  - Possessing the abilities presented in the book to an adequate degree factors heavily into older adults' overall health and well-being
  - Older adults who are in good health feel younger than their chronological age, while those in poor health feel the opposite
  - Rewards of aging include mastering professional skills and hobbies, gaining confidence, and enjoying rich relationships with loved ones, friends, and colleagues
- Theoretical Perspectives:
  - No clear-cut theory has emerged to explain the underlying causes of age-related cognitive-linguistic changes
  - It may be impossible for one theory to account for the various changes
  - Age-related cognitive theories can overlap
  - Inhibition Deficit:
    - ○ Aging weakens inhibitory processes, making it more difficult for older adults to suppress irrelevant information
  - Transmission Deficit:
    - ○ Age-related cognitive changes occur because memory connections are weakened, leading to poorer activation of the target information
  - Cognitive Slowing:
    - ○ Encompasses slower processing speed, reduced attentional abilities, and reduced working memory abilities
  - Reduced Resources, Reduced Working Memory:
    - ○ Older adults have fewer processing resources available to them than younger adults do, causing deficits when these resources are exceeded
  - Neurobiological Changes:
    - ○ Cognitive declines in normal aging result from reductions in prefrontal cortex function and dopamine

Discussion Questions

1. Why is chronological age typically reported when physical age takes one's overall health into consideration?
2. Does your definition of a "healthy" adult change if you know someone's chronological age? Why?
3. What are ways in which normal aging adults can strengthen memory connections?
4. Some benefits to aging are listed in the book. What are some other benefits to aging? Provide personal examples from your life.

References

Abraham, J. D., & Hansson, R. O. (1995). Successful aging at work: An applied study of selection, optimization, and compensation through impression management. *Journal of Gerontology: Psychological Sciences and Social Sciences, 50B,* 94–103.

Adams, C., Smith, M. C., Pasupathi, M., & Vitolo, L. (2002). Social context effects on story recall in older and younger women: Does the listener make a difference? *Journal of Gerontology: Psychological Sciences, 57B,* 28–40.

Adams, R. G., & Blieszner, R. (1995). Aging well with family and friends. *American Behavioral Scientist, 39,* 209–225.

American Speech-Language-Hearing Association. (2005). *Evidence-based practice in communication disorders* [Position statement]. Retrieved July 14, 2009, from www.asha.org/docs/html/PS2005-00221.html

Anderson, J. A. (1983). A spreading activation theory of memory. *Journal of Verbal Learning and Verbal Behavior, 22,* 261–295.

Anderson, J. D. (2007). Phonological neighborhood and word frequency effects in the stuttered disfluencies of children who stutter. *Journal of Speech, Language, and Hearing Research, 50,* 229–247.

Arnsten, A. F., Cai, J. X., Steere, J. C., & Goldman-Rakic, P. S. (1995). Dopamine D2 receptor mechanisms contribute to age-related cognitive decline: The effects of quinpirole on memory and motor function in monkeys. *Journal of Neurosciences, 15,* 3429–3439.

Baddeley, A. (2003). Working memory: Looking back and looking forward. *Nature Reviews Neuroscience, 4,* 829–839.

Braver, T. S., Barch, D. M., Keys, B. A., Carter, C. S., Cohen, J. D., Kaye, J. A. et al. (2001). Context processing in older adults: Evidence for a theory relating cognitive control to neurobiology in healthy aging. *Journal of Experimental Psychology, 4,* 746–763.

Brown, R., & McNeill, D. (1966). The "tip-of-the-tongue" phenomenon. *Journal of Verbal Learning and Verbal Behavior, 5,* 325–337.

Buckner, R. L., Head, D., & Lustig, C. (2006). Brain changes in aging: A lifespan perspective. In E. Bialystok & F. I. M. Craik (Eds.), *Lifespan cognition: Mechanisms of change* (pp. 27–43). New York: Oxford University Press.

Buckner, R. L., Kelley, W. H., & Petersen, S. E. (1999). Frontal cortex contributes to human memory formation. *Nature Neuroscience, 4,* 311–314.

Burda, A. N. (2007). *Communication changes in healthy aging adults.* Adele Whitenack Davis Research in Gerontology Award, University of Northern Iowa.

Burda, A. N. (2008). *Healthy aging adults' performance on tests of cognition.* Adele Whitenack Davis Research in Gerontology Award, University of Northern Iowa.

Burke, D. M., MacKay, D. G., Worthley, J. S., & Wade, E. (1991). On the tip of the tongue: What causes word finding failures in young and older adults? *Journal of Memory and Language, 30,* 542–579.

Caplan, D., & Waters, G. S. (1999). Verbal working memory and sentence comprehension. *Behavioral and Brain Sciences, 22,* 77–126.

Carlson, M. C., Fried, L. P., Xue, Q. L., Bandeen-Roche, K., Zeger, S. L., & Brandt, J. (1999). Association between executive attention and physical functional performance in community-dwelling older women. *Journal of Gerontology: Social Sciences, 54B,* S262–S270.

Cerella, J. (1985). Information processing rates in the elderly. *Psychological Bulletin, 98,* 67–83.

Cerella, J. (1990). Aging and information processing rate. In J. E. Birren & K. W. Schaie (Eds.), *Handbook of the psychology of aging* (3rd ed.) (pp. 201–221). New York: Academic Press.

Cohn, N. B., Dustman, R. E., & Bradford, D. C. (1984). Age-related decrements in Stroop color test performance. *Journal of Clinical Psychology, 40,* 1244–1250.

Collie, A., Shafiq-Antonacci, R., Maruff, P., Tyler, P., & Currie, J. (1999). Norms and the effects of demographic variables on neuropsychological battery for use in healthy ageing Australian populations. *Australian and New Zealand Journal of Psychiatry, 33,* 568–575.

Connelly, S. L., Hasher, L., & Zacks, R. T. (1991). Age and reading: The impact of distraction. *Psychology and Aging, 6,* 533–541.

Connor, L. T. (2001). Memory in old age: Patterns of decline and perseveration. *Seminars in Speech and Language, 22,* 117–125.

Constantinidou, F., & Baker, S. (2002). Stimulus modality and verbal learning performance in normal aging. *Brain and Language, 82,* 293–311.

Craik, F. I. M. (2000). Age-related changes in human memory. In D. Park & N. Schwarz (Eds.), *Cognitive aging: A primer* (pp. 75–92). Philadelphia: Psychology Press.

Davis, P., & Wright, E. A. (1977). A new method for measuring cranial cavity volume and its application to the assessment of cerebral atrophy at autopsy. *Neuropathology and Applied Neurobiology, 3,* 341–358.

De Beni, R., Palladino, P., Borella, E., & Lo Presti, S. (2003). Reading comprehension and aging: Does an age-related difference necessarily mean impairment? *Aging Clinical and Experimental Research, 15,* 67–76.

Ericsson, K. A., & Kintsch, W. (1995). Long-term working memory. *Psychological Review, 102,* 211–245.

Federmeier, K. D., Van Petten, C., Schwartz, T. J., & Kutas, M. (2003). Sounds, words, sentences: Age-related changes across several levels of processing. *Psychology and Aging, 18,* 858–872.

Fletcher, P. C., & Henson, R. N. A. (2001). Frontal lobes and human memory: Insights from functional neuroimaging. *Brain, 124,* 849–881.

Gana, K., Alaphilippe, D., & Bailly, N. (2004). Positive illusions and mental and physical health in later life. *Aging and Mental Health, 8,* 58–64.

Gollan, T., & Silverberg, N. (2001). Tip-of-the-tongue states in Hebrew-English bilinguals. *Bilingualism: Language and Cognition, 4,* 63–83.

Gordon-Salant, S., & Fitzgibbons, P. J. (1999). Profile of auditory temporal processing in older adults. *Journal of Speech, Language, and Hearing Research, 42,* 300–311.

Grady, C. L., McIntosh, A. R., Horwitz, B., Maisog, J. M., Ungerleider, L. G., Mentis, M. J., et al. (1995). Age-related reductions in human recognition memory due to impaired encoding. *Science*, 269, 218–221.

Hasher, L., & Zacks, R. T. (1988). Working memory, comprehension, and aging: A review and a new view. In G. H. Bower (Ed.), *The psychology of learning and motivation* (vol. 22, pp. 193–225). San Diego, CA: Academic Press.

Haug, H., & Eggers, R. (1991). Morphometry of the human cortex cerebri and corpus striatum during aging. *Neurobiology of Aging*, 12, 336–338.

Humes, L. E. (1996). Speech understanding in the elderly. *Journal of the American Academy of Audiology*, 7, 161–167.

Hutchinson, E. D. (2008). Middle adulthood. In E. Hutchinson (Ed.), *Dimensions of human behavior: The changing life course* (pp. 321–369). Thousand Oaks, CA: Sage Publications.

James, L. E. (2004). Meeting Mr. Farmer versus meeting a farmer: Specific effects of aging on learning proper names. *Psychology and Aging*, 19, 515–522.

James, L. E., & Burke, D. M. (2000). Phonological priming effects on word retrieval and tip-of-the-tongue experiences in young and older adults. *Journal of Experimental Psychology: Learning, Memory, and Cognition*, 26, 1378–1391.

James, L. E., Burke, D. M., Austin, A., & Hulme, E. (1998). Production and perception of "verbosity" in younger and older adults. *Psychological Aging*, 13, 355–367.

Kemper, S. (1986). Imitation of complex syntactic constructions by elderly adults. *Applied Psycholinguistics*, 7, 277–288.

Kemper, S. (2006). Language in adulthood. In E. Bialystok & F. I. M. Craik (Eds.), *Lifespan cognition: Mechanisms of change* (pp. 223–238). New York: Oxford University Press.

Kemper, S., Anagnopoulos, C., Lyons, K., & Heberlein, W. (1994). Speech accommodations to dementia. *Journal of Gerontology: Psychological Sciences*, 49, P223–P230.

Kemper, S., Herman, R. E., & Lian, C. H. (2003). The costs of doing two things at once for young and older adults: Talking while walking, finger tapping, and ignoring speech or noise. *Psychology and Aging*, 18, 181–192.

Kemper, S., Marquis, J., & Thompson, M. (2001). Longitudinal changes in language production: Effects of aging and dementia on grammatical complexity and propositional content. *Psychology and Aging*, 16, 600–614.

Kemper, S., & Sumner, A. (2001). The structure of verbal abilities in young and older adults. *Psychology and Aging*, 16, 312–322.

Li, S.-C., & Lindenberger, U. (1999). Cross-level unification: A computational exploration of the link between deterioration of neurotransmitter systems and dedifferentiation of cognitive abilities in old age. In L.-G. Nilsson & H. J. Markowitsch (Eds.), *Cognitive neuroscience of memory* (pp. 103–146). Toronto, ON: Hogrefe & Huber.

Li, S.-C., Lindenberger, U., & Frensch, P. A. (2000). Unifying cognitive aging: From neuromodulation to representation to cognition. *Neurocomputing*, 32–33, 879–890.

Li, S.-C., Lindenberger, U., & Sikstrom, S. (2001). Aging cognition: From neuromodulation to representation to cognition. *Trends in Cognitive Sciences*, 5, 479–486.

Light, L. L. (1991). Memory and aging: Four hypotheses in search of data. *Annual Review of Psychology*, 42, 333–376.

Little, D. M., Prentice, K. J., Darrow, A. W., & Wingfield, A. (2005). Listening to spoken text: Adult age differences as revealed by self-paced listening. *Experimental Aging Research*, 31, 313–330.

Logan, J. M., Sanders, A. L., Snyder, A. Z., Morris, J. C., & Buckner, R. L. (2002). Under-recruitment and nonselective recruitment: Dissociable neural mechanisms associated with aging. *Neuron*, 33, 827–840.

Logan, J. R., Ward, R., & Spitze, G. (1992). As old as you feel: Age identity in middle and later life. *Social Forces, 71*, 451–467.

MacKay, D. G., & James, L. E. (2001). Is cognitive aging all downhill? Current theory versus reality. *Human Development, 44*, 288–295.

MacKay, D. G., & James, L. E. (2004). Sequencing, speech production, and selective effects of aging on phonological and morphological speech errors. *Psychology and Aging, 19*, 93–107.

MacKinlay, E. (2006). *Spiritual growth and care in the fourth age of life.* Philadelphia: Jessica Kingsley Publishers.

Maylor, E. A. (1997). Proper name retrieval in old age: Converging evidence against disproportionate impairment. *Aging, Neuropsychology, and Cognition, 4*, 211–226.

Meijer, W. A., De Groot, R. H. M., Van Boxtel, M. P. J., Van Gerven, P. W. M., & Jolles, J. (2006). Verbal learning and aging: Combined effects of irrelevant speech, interstimulus interval, and education. *Journal of Gerontology: Psychological Sciences, 61B*, P285–P294.

Mortensen, L., Meyer, A. S., & Humphreys, G. W. (2006). Age-related effects on speech production: A review. *Language and Cognitive Processes, 21*, 238–290.

Moscovitch, M., & Wincour, G. (1995). Frontal lobes, memory, and aging. *Annals of the New York Academy of Sciences, 769*, 119–151.

Munson, B. (2007). Lexical access, lexical representation, and vowel articulation. In J. Cole & J. Hualde (Eds.), *Laboratory phonology 9* (pp. 201–228). New York: Mouton de Gruyter.

Myerson, J., Hale, S., Wagstaff, D., Poon, L. W., & Smith, G. A. (1990). The information loss model: A mathematical theory of age-related cognitive slowing. *Psychological Review, 97*, 475–487.

Nakamura, E., Moritani, T., & Kanetaka, A. (1989). Biological age versus physical fitness age. *European Journal of Applied Physiology and Occupational Physiology, 58*, 778–785.

Nyberg, L., Sandblom, J., Jones, S., Stigsdotter-Neely, A., Magnus-Petersson, K., Ingvar, M. et al. (2003). Neural correlates of train-related memory improvement in adulthood and aging. *Proceedings of the National Academy of Sciences, USA, 100*, 13728–13733.

Parkin, A. J., & Java, R. I. (1999). Deterioration of frontal lobe function in normal aging: Influences of fluid intelligence versus perceptual speed. *Neuropsychology, 13*, 539–545.

Peel, N., Bartlett, H., & McClure, R. (2004). Healthy ageing: How is it defined and measured? *Australasian Journal on Ageing, 23*, 115–119.

Perfect, T. (1997). Memory aging as frontal lobe dysfunction. In M. A. Conway (Ed.), *Cognitive models of memory* (pp. 315–339). Cambridge, MA: MIT Press.

Pichora-Fuller, M. K., Schneider, B. A., & Daneman, M. (1995). How young and old adults listen to and remember speech in noise. *Journal of the Acoustical Society of America, 97*, 593–608.

Rabbitt, P., & Anderson, M. (2006). The lacunae of loss? Aging and the differentiation of cognitive abilities. In E. Bialystok & F. I. M. Craik (Eds.), *Lifespan cognition: Mechanisms of change* (pp. 331–343). New York: Oxford University Press.

Rastle, K. G., & Burke, D. M. (1996). Priming the tip of the tongue: Effects of prior processing on word retrieval in young and older adults. *Journal of Memory and Language, 35*, 586–605.

Reilly, S., Douglas, J., & Oates, J. (2004). *Evidence-based practice in speech pathology.* London: Whurr.

Salat, D. H., Kaye, J. A., & Janowsky, J. S. (1999). Prefrontal gray and white matter volumes in healthy aging and Alzheimer's disease. *Archives of Neurology, 56*, 338–344.

Salthouse, T. A. (1985). *The theory of cognitive aging.* Amsterdam: North-Holland.

Salthouse, T. A. (1988a). Resource-reduction interpretations of cognitive aging. *Developmental Review, 8,* 238–272.

Salthouse, T. A. (1988b). The role of processing resources in cognitive ageing. In M. L. Howe & C. J. Brainerd (Eds.), *Cognitive development in adulthood* (pp. 185–239). New York: Springer-Verlag.

Salthouse, T. A. (1990). Working memory as a processing resource in cognitive aging. *Developmental Review, 10,* 101–124.

Salthouse, T. A. (1996). Constraints on theories of cognitive aging. *Psychology and Aging,* 3, 287–299.

Salthouse, T. A., Kausler, D., & Saults, J. S. (1988). Utilization of path-analytic procedures to investigate the role of processing resources in cognitive aging. *Psychology and Aging,* 3, 158–166.

Salthouse, T. A., & Lichty, W. (1985). Tests of the neural noise hypothesis of age-related cognitive change. *Journal of Gerontology, 40,* 443–450.

Schmitt, J. F. (1983). The effects of time compression and time expansion on passage comprehension by elderly listeners. *Journal of Speech and Hearing Research, 26,* 373–377.

Schneider, B. A., Daneman, M., Murphy, D. R., & Kwong-See, S. (2000). Listening to discourse in distracting settings: The effects of aging. *Psychology and Aging, 15,* 110–125.

Schwartz, B. L. (2002). *Tip-of-the-tongue states: Phenomenology, mechanism, and lexical retrieval.* Mahwah, NJ: Lawrence Erlbaum Associates.

Shadden, B. B., & Toner, M. A. (1997). Introduction: The continuum of life functions. In B. B. Shadden & M. A. Toner (Eds.), *Aging and communication: For clinicians by clinicians* (pp. 3–17). Austin, TX: Pro-Ed.

Shankle, R. S., & Amen, D. G. (2005). *Preventing Alzheimer's: Ways to prevent, detect, diagnose, treat, and even halt Alzheimer's disease and other causes of memory loss.* New York: Penguin.

Skirbekk, V. (2003). *Age and individual productivity: A literature survey.* MPIDR, Working Paper No. 2003–028.

Sommers, M. S. (1996). The structural organization of the mental lexicon and its contributions to age-related declines in spoken and word recognition. *Psychology and Aging, 11,* 333–341.

Sommers, M. S., & Danielson, S. M. (1999). Inhibitory processes and spoken word recognition in young and older adults: The interaction of lexical competition and semantic context. *Psychology and Aging, 14,* 458–472.

Spieler, D. H., & Balota, D. A. (2000). Factors influencing word naming in younger and older adults. *Psychology and Aging, 15,* 253–258.

Stephens, N. (1991). Cognitive aging: A useful concept for advertising? *Journal of Advertising, 20,* 37–48.

Stine, E. A. L., & Wingfield, A. (1987). Process and strategy in memory for speech among younger and older adults. *Psychology and Aging, 2,* 272–279.

Stine-Morrow, E. A. L., Gagne, D., Morrow, D. G., & DeWall, B. (2004). Age differences in rereading. *Memory and Cognition, 32,* 696–710.

Stine-Morrow, E. A. L., Loveless, M. K., & Soederberg, L. M. (1996). Resource allocation in on-line reading by younger and older adults. *Psychology and Aging, 11,* 475–486.

Stine-Morrow, E. A. L., Miller, L. M. S., & Leno, I. R. (2001). Aging and resource allocation to narrative text. *Aging, Neuropsychology, and Cognition, 8,* 36–53.

Suhara, T., Fukuda, H., Inoue, O., Itoh, T., Suzuki, K., Yamasaki, T. et al. (1991). Age-related changes in human D1 dopamine receptors measured by positron emission tomography. *Psychopharmacology, 103,* 41–45.

Thornton, R., & Light, L. L. (2006). Language comprehension and production in normal aging. In J. E. Birren & K. W. Schaie (Eds.), *Handbook of the psychology of aging* (6th ed., pp. 261–287). San Diego, CA: Elsevier.

Tun, P. A., O'Kane, G., & Wingfield, A. (2002). Distraction by competing speech in young and older adult listeners. *Psychology and Aging, 17,* 453–467.

van Rooij, J. C. G. M., & Plomp, M. (1990). Auditive and cognitive factors in speech perception in elderly listeners. II: Multivariate analyses. *Journal of the Acoustical Society of America, 88,* 2611–2624.

Vitevitch, M. S., & Sommers, M. S. (2003). The facilitative influence of phonological similarity and neighborhood frequency in speech production in younger and older adults. *Memory and Cognition, 31,* 491–504.

Waters, G. S., & Caplan, D. (1996). The capacity theory of sentence comprehension. Critique of Just and Carpenter (1992). *Psychological Review, 103,* 761–772.

Waters, G. S., & Caplan, D. (2001). Age, working memory and on-line syntactic processing in sentence comprehension. *Psychology and Aging, 16,* 128–144.

Waters, G. S., & Caplan, D. (2005). The relationship between age, processing speed, working memory capacity, and language comprehension. *Memory, 13,* 403–413.

West, R. L. (1996). An application of prefrontal cortex function theory to cognitive aging. *Psychological Bulletin, 120,* 272–292.

White, K. K., & Abrams, L. (1999, November). *The role of syllable phonology and aging in priming tip-of-the-tongue resolution.* Poster session presented at annual meeting of the Psychonomic Society, Los Angeles, CA.

Whiting, W. L., Madden, D. J., Langley, L. K., Denny, L. L., Turkington, T. G., Provenzale, J. M. et al. (2003). Lexical and sublexical components of age-related changes in neural activation during visual word identification. *Journal of Cognitive Neuroscience, 15,* 475–487.

Wingfield, A., & Ducharme, J. L. (1999). Effects of age and passage difficulty on listening-rate preferences for time-altered speech. *Journal of Gerontology: Psychological Sciences and Social Sciences, 54B,* 199–202.

Wingfield, A., Lahar, C. J., & Stine, E. L. (1989). Age and decision strategies in running memory for speech: Effects of prosody and linguistic structure. *Journal of Gerontology: Psychological Sciences, 44,* P106–P113.

Wingfield, A., Tun, P. A., & Rosen, M. J. (1995). Age differences in vertical and reconstructive recall of syntactically and randomly segmented speech. *Journal of Gerontology: Psychological Sciences, 50B,* P257–P266.

Worrall, L. E., & Hickson, L. M., (2003). *Communication disability in aging: From prevention to intervention.* Clifton Park, NY: Thomson Delmar Learning.

Zacks, R. T., & Hasher, L. (1988). Capacity theory and the processing of inferences. In L. L. Light & D. M. Burke (Eds.), *Language, memory, and aging* (pp. 154–170). Cambridge: Cambridge University Press.

Zacks, R. T., & Hasher, L. (1997). Cognitive gerontology and attentional inhibition: A reply to Burke and McDowd. *Journal of Gerontology: Psychological Sciences, 52B,* 274–283.

Chapter **2**

Cognition

Angela N. Burda, PhD, CCC-SLP

Introduction

Cognition is one small word that conveys a host of multifaceted abilities. Having adequate cognitive skills lets us go through our day without having to "think" about automatic activities, such as brushing our teeth or getting dressed (Rogers, 2000). We can then focus our resources on specific tasks, such as preparing for a work presentation or driving in bad weather (Rogers, 2000). Intact cognition also allows us to pay attention to what someone is saying despite a noisy background, plan for the day ahead, remember to stop by the grocery store to pick up ingredients for that night's dinner, and make alternate dinner plans when the needed ingredients are unavailable.

The broad areas of cognition are attention, memory, executive functions, and problem solving. Attention permits us to focus on certain information for processing while ignoring irrelevant information (Enns & Trick, 2006). Memory allows individuals to retain, recall, and manipulate information (Duckworth, Iezzi, & O'Donohue, 2008; Park & Payer, 2006). Executive functions are composed of such abilities as planning, organizing, initiating, and stopping behaviors (Posner, 2008). Problem solving lets us generate solutions for given situations (Kennedy & Coelho, 2005). These various skills can overlap and also underlie language abilities. For example, if we pay close attention and remember what the speaker is saying during a workshop, it is more likely that we can better formulate questions to ask. There are also various theoretical perspectives to keep in mind regarding age-related cognitive changes (see Chapter 1 on theoretical perspectives).

This chapter discusses what aging adults' cognitive abilities generally should be, factors that can negatively affect older adults' cognition, signs that may warrant referral to a speech-language pathologist or other medical professionals, and strategies that can foster aging adults' cognitive abilities. A list of "Quick Facts" at the end of the chapter summarizes important points.

Older Adults' General Cognitive Abilities

Speech-language pathologists (SLPs) frequently assess their patients' cognition. Assessment tools generally divide cognition into broad areas, such as attention and memory, although some tests further assess areas like organization, immediate memory, and recall of general information (Bayles & Tomoeda, 1993; Helm-Estabrooks, 2001; Ross-Swain & Fogle, 1996). Tests may be arranged in a hierarchical manner, beginning with items requiring short, simple responses and progressing to lengthier, more complex items (Ross-Swain, 1996). Several of the commercially available cognitive tests for adults involve such tasks as repeating strings of numbers or words of increasing length, conducting visual searches, performing symbol cancellation tasks, and retelling stories both immediately after hearing them and following a delay. Other items assess the person's abilities to respond to orientation questions, provide solutions to problematic situations, verbally generate items in a given category within one minute, and answer open-ended questions related to long-term memory, such as where the capitol of the United States is, and who the first president was (Bayles & Tomoeda, 1993; Helm-Estabrooks, 2001; Ross-Swain, 1996).

Although a great deal of research has been conducted on neurologically intact older adults' cognitive abilities, studies have not necessarily evaluated clinical tasks found in tests used by SLPs, such as those previously mentioned. Not all tests on cognition have systematically included aging adults as part of the standardization process. Tests that have included older adults as part of the normative sample do not necessarily document age-specific performance in the assessment manuals (Helm-Estabrooks, 2001). Some exceptions exist, and information found in test manuals, coupled with empirical data in the literature, can provide a general guide of what the normal cognitive abilities are for neurologically intact older adults.

In the development of the *Arizona Battery for Communication Disorders of Dementia* (ABCD; Bayles & Tomoeda, 1993), neurologically intact older adults were included as a separate control group, with a mean age of 70.44 years. Subtests that assess cognition include Mental Status, Generative Naming Semantic Category, Story Retelling–Immediate, Story Retelling–Delayed, and Word Learning. The Mental Status subtest asks orientation and biographical questions, such as "In what city are we?" and "In what month do we celebrate Independence Day?" Older adults in the normative sample received a mean score of 12.8 items correct (SD = 0.6) out of a total of 13 possible, or 98% correct, which is similar to the mean score of the young adult control group (M = 12.9, SD = 0.3). Although the ABCD's Generative Naming Semantic Category subtest can also be viewed as a verbal-expression task, categorization tasks are frequently included as part of cognitive batteries. This subtest asks persons to name as many different items as possible in a given category (modes of transportation) within one minute. Older adults in the normative sample named a mean of 11.4 items within one minute, while younger adults generated an average of 13.4 items.

For the ABCD's Story Retelling subtests, patients retell a story right after hearing it and then following a delay. The immediate retelling subtest occurs early in the test; the delayed retelling is the last task of the entire test. Fifteen subtests are administered between the two subtests. Patients are prompted at the end of the immediate retelling subtest to remember the information because they will be asked about it later. The story is about a woman who is unaware that she lost her wallet while shopping. She then receives a call from a little girl who found the wallet. Scores are calculated based on patients' reporting correct informational units (e.g., "lady," "her wallet").

For the Story Retelling–Immediate subtest, older adults in the normative sample recalled an average of 14 information units (SD = 2.8) out of a total of 17 information units possible, or 82% correct. Young adults recalled nearly 15 information units (88% correct). On the Story Retelling–Delayed subtest, the older adults recalled an average of 12.4 information units (SD = 4.5), or 73% correct. Scores for the Story Retelling–Immediate subtest do not differ significantly between neurologically intact young and old adults. However, performance does differ between the two age groups on the Story Retelling–Delayed subtest. In this subtest, older adults recalled roughly 12 information units, while young adults recalled approximately 15 information units (Bayles & Tomoeda, 1993).

Three separate scores are obtained in the Word Learning subtest: Word Learning–Free Recall, Word Learning–Total Recall, and Word Learning–Recognition. Individuals are presented with a series of pages, each with four words on it (e.g., emerald, head, trumpet, shark). Persons identify the word that matches a brief description of each, such as "the precious stone" or "the fish." For Free Recall, individuals count from 1 to 20 after the presentation of all 16 words (i.e., four pages with four words per page) and then recall as many words as they can in two minutes. For Cued Recall, the SLP provides cues for any missed items by stating their categories (e.g., "the precious stone"). The Free Recall and Cued Recall scores are combined to give the Total Recall score. Recognition scores are obtained by showing patients 48 cards, each with a printed word on it, and then asking them to state whether or not the words appeared on the previously shown pages. For the Word Learning–Free Recall section, older adults received a mean score of 7.6 (SD = 2.5) out of 16 possible, or 48% correct. Young adults, however, received a mean score of 10.4 (SD = 2.1), or 65% correct. On the Word Learning–Total Recall section, older adults had a mean score of 15.1 (SD = 1.2) out of 16 possible, or 94% correct, which does not differ significantly from the mean score of the young adults, 15.7 items (SD = 0.6). On the Word Learning–Recognition portion, older adults received a mean score of 46.6 (SD = 2.5) out of 48 cards, or 97% correct, which is fairly similar to the mean score of the younger adults, 47.8 (SD = 0.6) (Bayles & Tomoeda, 1993).

The *Ross Information Processing Assessment–Geriatric* (RIPA-G; Ross-Swain & Fogle, 1996) specifically tests older adults' cognition. Fifty neurologically intact adults aged 65 to 94 (M_{age} = 79) served as a control group. Subtests target several areas, including: immediate and delayed memory, various types of orientation (e.g., spatial orientation, orientation to the environment), recall of general information, problem solving, thought organization, and abstract and concrete reasoning. A total of 30 points is possible for each subtest. Older adults scored a mean of 27.6, or 92% accuracy, on the Immediate Recall subtest. Sample items on that subtest include digit-span recall (e.g., 9-3-7-5-8) and following directions (e.g., "Close your eyes and raise your hand"). Aging adults recalled information for the Recent Memory subtest (e.g., stating the first thing they did that morning or where they spent most of the previous day) with a mean score of 28.6, or 95% accuracy. On the Organization subtest, persons list as many items in a category (e.g., foods) as they can within one minute and name a category when given specific members (e.g., dogs, cats, and horses). Older persons scored a mean of 28.1 (94% accuracy) on this subtest and completed the remaining seven subtests with mean minimum accuracy scores of at least 29 points, or 97% accuracy. The examiner's manual from another test developed by Ross-Swain (1996) to assess cognition, the *Ross Information Processing Assessment*, 2nd edition (RIPA-2), does not contain normative data for healthy older adults.

Research also has been conducted on older adults' cognitive abilities. Recently, Burda (2008) sought to provide additional data in terms of how well healthy, aging adults perform on cognitive tests commonly administered by SLPs. Thirty adults aged 65 and older were divided into three age categories: Young-Old (ages 65–74; $M_{age} = 72.2$ years, $SD = 1.6$), Middle-Old (ages 75–84; $M_{age} = 79.1$ years, $SD = 2.8$), and Old-Old (ages 85+; $M_{age} = 87.9$ years, $SD = 3.1$). Ten participants were in each age group. All participants completed three cognitive tests: the RIPA-G (Ross-Swain & Fogle, 1996), the RIPA-2 (Ross-Swain, 1996), and the Cognitive Linguistic Quick Test (CLQT; Helm-Estabrooks, 2001). Descriptive results and outcomes from a series of one-factor analyses of variance (ANOVA) using the Bonferroni correction for multiple comparisons are included below. Note that 30 is the highest possible raw score for all subtests of the RIPA-G and RIPA-2.

In most cases, the Old-Old group had the lowest mean scores on the RIPA-G (Ross-Swain & Fogle, 1996), except for Subtest IV, in which the Young-Old had the lowest score (**Table 2-1**). The Middle-Old group generally had the highest mean scores. Overall, all age groups generally had high mean scores, which is similar to what Ross-Swain (1996) reported in the RIPA-G's examiner's manual. Statistically significant performance differences occurred on Subtest VIII, $F (2, 27) = 4.14$, $p \leq 0.03$.

Table 2-1

Mean Performance for the RIPA-G

Subtest	Young-Old		Middle-Old		Old-Old	
	M	SD	M	SD	M	SD
I: Immediate Memory	27.11	2.74	28.20	1.99	26.30	3.40
II: Recent Memory	29.56	0.84	29.60	0.84	28.70	1.25
III: Temporal Orientation	29.78	0.48	30.00	0.00	29.00	1.25
IV: Spatial Orientation	29.78	0.63	30.00	0.00	29.90	0.32
V: Orientation to Environment	30.00	0.00	30.00	0.00	30.00	0.00
VI: Recall of General Info	28.89	1.63	29.50	1.08	28.50	2.51
VII: Problem Solving and Abstract Reasoning	30.00	0.00	29.90	0.32	29.80	0.63
VIII: Organization of Info	29.44	0.84	29.50	0.71	28.10	1.79
IX: Auditory Processing and Comprehension	29.56	1.49	30.00	0.00	29.20	1.48
X: Problem Solving and Concrete Reasoning	29.78	1.08	29.80	0.63	29.40	0.97
XI: Naming Common Objects	30.00	0.00	30.00	0.00	29.80	0.63
XII: Functional Oral Reading	30.00	0.00	30.00	0.00	30.00	0.00

Source: Burda (2008).

Table 2-2

Mean Performance for the RIPA-2

Subtest	Young-Old M	Young-Old SD	Middle-Old M	Middle-Old SD	Old-Old M	Old-Old SD
I: Immediate Memory	26.40	3.57	23.90	3.73	20.60	2.67
II: Recent Memory–Temporal	29.50	1.08	29.60	0.70	27.70	1.49
III: Orientation (Recent Memory)	29.80	0.42	30.00	0.00	28.30	2.75
IV: Temporal Orientation (Remote Memory)	29.30	1.06	29.10	1.29	28.70	1.49
V: Spatial Orientation	30.00	0.00	30.00	0.00	29.80	0.63
VI: Orientation to Environment	29.90	0.32	29.90	0.32	29.60	1.26
VII: Recall of General Information	28.30	2.21	28.40	1.96	26.60	4.03
VIII: Problem Solving and Abstract Reasoning	29.80	0.63	30.00	0.00	28.80	2.82
IX: Organization	27.40	1.78	28.30	1.25	25.00	2.62
X: Auditory Processing and Retention	29.50	1.08	29.90	0.32	28.30	1.64

Source: Burda (2008).

As can be seen in **Table 2-2**, the Old-Old group consistently had the lowest mean scores on the RIPA-2 (Ross-Swain, 1996), and with the exception of Subtest I, all age groups had high overall mean scores on this test. Statistically significant performance differences occurred on several subtests: II, F $(2, 27) = 7.72, p \leq 0.002$; III, F $(2, 27) = 5.23$, $p \leq 0.01$; VI, F $(2, 27) = 3.74, p \leq 0.05$; IX, F $(2, 27) = 5.61, p \leq 0.05$; and X, F $(2, 27) = 4.37, p \leq 0.05$.

All groups earned the highest possible score on the Personal Facts and Confrontation Naming subtests (**Table 2-3**). In the remaining CLQT (Helm-Estabrooks, 2001) subtests, those in the Old-Old group had the lowest mean performance scores. Statistically significant performance differences occurred on the subtests of Clock Drawing, F $(2, 27) = 9.01, p \leq 0.001$; Symbol Trails, F $(2, 27) = 5.93, p \leq 0.007$; and Generative Naming, F $(2, 27) = 6.41, p \leq 0.005$.

Scores obtained from the subtests of the CLQT are also used to help determine scores for the cognitive domains. As with the subtests on the CLQT, participants in the Old-Old group also had the lowest mean performance on the domains (**Table 2-4**). In fact, this age group had scores that would not be considered within normal limits for the domains of Attention, Memory, and Language. There were statistically

Table 2-3

Mean Performance for Subtests of the CLQT

Subtest	HPS	Young-Old		Middle-Old		Old-Old	
		M	SD	M	SD	M	SD
Personal Facts	8	8.00	0.00	8.00	0.00	8.00	0.00
Symbol Cancellation	12	10.70	3.77	11.90	0.31	9.60	3.56
Confrontation Naming	10	10.00	0.00	10.00	0.00	10.00	0.00
Clock Drawing	13	12.10	1.10	12.90	0.31	10.80	1.54
Story Retelling	10	7.50	2.06	7.60	1.83	5.70	2.49
Symbol Trails	10	10.00	0.00	9.00	2.16	7.20	2.34
Generative Naming	8	6.55	1.17	6.40	0.69	4.90	1.37
Design Memory	6	4.90	1.19	5.30	0.82	4.50	1.17
Mazes	8	6.35	2.56	6.70	1.58	5.25	2.39
Design Generation	8	6.00	1.69	5.90	1.28	5.10	2.02

Abbreviation: HPS = highest possible score
Source: Burda (2008).

Table 2-4

Mean Performance for Domains of the CLQT

Domain	WNL	Young-Old		Middle-Old		Old-Old	
		M	SD	M	SD	M	SD
Attention	175–215	182.50	47.43	192.60	14.56	154.50	35.25
Memory	158–185	156.50	21.99	161.00	13.92	140.10	25.06
Executive Functions	18–40	30.85	7.00	28.30	3.72	22.45	4.18
Language	30–37	32.00	3.00	34.10	6.64	28.60	3.37
Visuospatial Skills	72–105	86.50	17.00	87.00	10.57	72.45	11.32

Abbreviation: WNL = within normal limits (according to the examiner's manual)
Source: Burda (2008).

significant differences on the domains of Executive Functions, F $(2, 27)$ = 6.93, $p \leq 0.004$; Language, F $(2, 27)$ = 3.59, $p \leq 0.04$; and Visuospatial Skills, F $(2, 27)$ = 3.87, $p \leq 0.03$.

Although this study contained a small sample size, all participant groups generally had high scores on both the RIPA-G (Ross-Swain & Fogle, 1996) and the RIPA-2 (Ross-Swain, 1996). Compared with the results from the RIPA-G and the RIPA-2, participants' performance on the CLQT (Helm-Estabrooks, 2001) is more difficult to interpret. As with the previous two tests, those in the Old-Old age group generally had the lowest performance scores on the CLQT. In some cases, these scores fell below those that are considered within normal limits on the CLQT domains. Despite this, all participants were healthy and lived independently. Thus, such scores should be viewed with caution; more research needs to be conducted with a larger sample size.

Several other studies have also examined aging and cognition. Those in the areas of attention and memory frequently specify the particular type of these abilities (e.g., selective attention, episodic memory). Selective attention refers to the ability to focus on important information while ignoring irrelevant information (Kramer & Kray, 2006) and is often measured by having individuals visually search for a particular target letter in a list of letters. In focused attention, individuals know where the target is, but distracting information is also present (Rogers, 2000). Attending a movie in a crowded theater is a good illustration of this skill. The screen location stays the same while distractions such as people talking and those trying to find a seat must be filtered out. Focused attention requires intense concentration involving a search through a complex visual field. For example, when individuals come back from getting popcorn to have during a movie, they must scan through the other people in the theater to find their seat (Rogers, 2000). Sustained attention refers to actively processing information over an extended period of time. Real-world examples include assembly-line workers searching for faulty items or parents listening for an infant's cry (Rogers, 2000). Divided attention is the ability to perform more than one task at the same time. Driving a car, for example, requires attention to many pieces of information, such as lane tracking and watching for other vehicles or pedestrians (Kramer & Kray, 2006).

Older adults are slower than younger adults on selective attention visual searches, particularly if they have to pay attention to more than one feature of the target (e.g., finding the red Xs in a field of green Xs and red Os; Plude & Doussard-Roosevelt, 1989), if the distractor letters are similar to the target (e.g., O vs. Q as opposed to O vs. T), or if they do not know where the target is located (Rogers, 2000). Extensive practice does not help their speed (Fisk & Rogers, 1991; Salthouse, 2000). Focused attention, however, remains relatively intact as long as the target is easily discernible (Riddle, 2007; Rogers, 2000). If the target is not easy to identify, its location is unknown, or a search requires attention to several features, older adults have greater difficulty focusing their attention (Rogers, 2000). Changes in sustained attention have not been clearly identified. Although some researchers have not found any age effects on sustained-attention tasks (Berardi, Parasuraman, & Haxby, 2001), others report that older adults have greater challenges with tasks that require detecting subtle changes, such as distinguishing between a 17-mm square and a 20-mm square (Giambra, 1993).

Researchers tend to use dual-task conditions to study divided attention. For example, participants are presented with word lists in which they judge whether or not an item is a word or nonword, and press a key on a keyboard when a randomly presented auditory tone is played (Simpson, Kellas, & Ferraro, 1999). Although older adults do as well as younger adults on simple divided attention tasks, such as walking and reciting the alphabet, they perform poorer when the activities are complex, such as walking and reciting alternating letters of the alphabet (Verghese, Buschke, Viola, Hall, Kuslansky, & Lipton, 2002). Older adults react slower, in some cases up to 53% slower, in processing incoming stimuli, coordinating, and carrying out the required responses (Kramer, Humphrey, Larish, Logan, & Strayer, 1994; Simpson et al., 1999). Older adults' speech also becomes slower, less fluent, and less complex while walking, tapping their fingers, or ignoring background noise (Kemper, Herman, & Lian, 2003).

Memory, similar to attention, is differentiated into specific abilities (Baddeley, 2003; Craik, 2000). Procedural memory refers to the learning and retention of various motor, cognitive, and academic abilities that have a significant automatic element associated with them, such as driving a car, setting the table, counting, and spelling (Craik, 2000). Working memory requires individuals to manipulate, store, and transform pieces of information (Baddeley, 2003). Mentally calculating the tip to leave at a restaurant is an example of this ability. In short-term memory, storage of information is temporary, assumed to have a limited capacity of seven chunks, and if attention is diverted to another task, the information originally stored there can become unavailable in a matter of seconds (Brown, 1958; Miller, 1956; Peterson & Peterson, 1959). More recently, others suggest that short-term memory has an even more limited capacity of three to five chunks of information (Cowan, 2001, 2008). Episodic memory is the ability to recall specific autobiographical events that have been experienced relatively recently, such as remembering a recent vacation (Zacks & Hasher, 2006). Prospective memory is the capability to carry out future events, and semantic memory refers to the store of general or factual knowledge that we possess (Craik, 2000; Duckworth et al., 2008). It is how we know that a dog is an animal but one that differs from a cat, or that a street differs from an interstate. Remote memory, which some may refer to as long-term memory, is the recall of events that happened to individuals when they were children or young adults (Craik, 2000), such as driving their first car, going to the high school state championship football game, and meeting their spouse. Its storage capacity is thought to be immense (Cowan, 2001; Ericsson & Kintsch, 1995).

Although memory abilities do decline in aging adults, it generally depends upon the specific memory task tested; some skills will show significant declines, while others will not (Craik, 2000). Procedural memory appears to remain intact in healthy older adults (Craik, 2000). This is not surprising, because people do not forget how to drive or count as they age. Working memory can have considerable age-related declines if more than a small amount of information needs to be manipulated (Craik, 2000; Connor, 2001). For example, aging adults can accurately copy a telephone number or transcribe a small amount of information from one part of a form to another (Craik, 2000). Older adults can have significant difficulty with lengthy or complex material, such as that involved in taking a telephone survey in which several answers must be kept in working memory (Craik, 2000). Some researchers report that a reduction in aging adults' working memory can lead to less grammatically complex language (Kemper & Sumner, 2001).

Older adults have reduced short-term and episodic memory (Ericsson & Kintsch, 1995; Naveh-Benjamin, Hussain, Guez, & Bar-On, 2003). It can be difficult to tease out the differences between the two because studies employ similar tasks and may use the terms somewhat interchangeably. Researchers often use immediate and delayed free recall of words, sentences, narrative stories, expository prose (e.g., newspaper articles), and pictures to test episodic memory and have reported poorer performance in older adults compared with young and middle-aged adults (Craik, 2000; Dobbs & Rule, 1989; Hultsch & Dixon, 1984; Kemper, 1987). Older adults also tend to do poorer on digit-span tasks compared with young and middle-aged adults (Jenkins, Myerson, Hale, & Fry, 1999). In a recent study, adults in different age groups recalled 15 nouns from the *Rey Auditory Verbal Learning Test* (Rey, 1964) that were presented over five successive trials (Davis, Small, Stern, Mayeux, Feldstein, & Keller, 2003). Adults aged 76–90 recalled 11 words after a 20-minute delay, those aged 61–75 remembered 12 words, and young and middle-aged adults recalled 14 words. Aging adults typically have difficulty remembering specific facts, remembering where and when they experienced a particular event or learned certain information, and making the connection of why someone's face is familiar (Craik, 2000). Not only can they have difficulty recalling newly learned information, they can forget that information more rapidly (Davis et al., 2003). Word-finding problems increase (Craik, 2000; Wierenga et al., 2006) and recalling names can be particularly challenging, even though older adults can recall biographical information, attributes, or the image of the person (Cohen & Faulkner, 1986; James, 2006).

Prospective memory is well maintained in older adults, possibly because they have established strategies such as taking notes or setting up a reminder system (Chasteen, Park, & Schwartz, 2009). Semantic memory also shows little decline with age (Hedden & Gabrieli, 2004; Light, 1992; Light & Burke, 1988; Salthouse, 1982). Recognition memory and word meaning knowledge remains intact (Craik & Jennings, 1992; Davis et al., 2003; Salthouse, 1991; Zacks, Hasher, & Li, 1999).

In remote memory, older adults may contrast their ability to easily recall salient experiences that happened to them as children or young adults with their difficulties in remembering recent information (Craik, 2000). This information has likely been activated many times over the course of several years and thus tends to not show significant decline (Craik, 2000). Skilled activities stored in long-term memory, such as expert performance seen in medical professionals or advanced chess players, also do not tend to show marked change over time (Ericsson & Kintsch, 1995).

Executive functions are needed to organize, initiate, and carry out a sequence of actions (Carlson, Fried, Xue, Bandeen-Roche, Zeger, & Brandt, 1999). Even a relatively easy task such as unlocking a door has several steps: picking up the key, inserting it into the lock, and turning the key until the door is unlocked (Carlson et al., 1999). Researchers have found that older adults have poor executive function performance on neuropsychological tests (Crawford & Channon, 2002). In contrast, their reasoning abilities tend to be preserved for real-life situations (Phillips & Della Salla, 1998). Unfortunately, many of the evaluations used by healthcare professionals do not necessarily indicate how age-related changes in executive functions may impact everyday activities, such as preparing meals or making phone calls (Carlson et al., 1999).

Some authors include problem solving as part of executive functioning abilities, while others discuss it as a separate topic. Regardless, successful problem solving requires individuals to take into account not only the facts of the situation but also the persons involved and their perspectives, the practicality of differing solutions, and the potential consequences of these solutions (Crawford & Channon, 2002). Older adults are quite effective in their problem-solving skills. Although they may generate fewer solutions than young adults, their solutions tend to be complex, flexible, and of high quality (Blanchard-Fields, Mienaltowski, & Baldi Seay, 2007; Crawford & Channon, 2002). Aging adults tend to use proactive strategies to solve instrumental problems, such as taking precautions to ensure their safety if a rash of burglaries occurs in their neighborhood (Blanchard-Fields, Chen, & Norris, 1997; Blanchard-Fields, Jahnke, & Camp, 1995; Cornelius & Capsi, 1987). On the other hand, they select passive emotion regulation strategies to deal with interpersonal problems, such as trying to figure out why friends are not coming to visit despite them wanting the company (Cornelius & Capsi, 1987). This selection of different strategies could result from older adults having had many opportunities to hone their problem-solving skills over their lifetime (Blanchard-Fields et al., 2007).

In summary, based on data from cognitive tests and research studies, older adults can accurately answer orientation and biographical questions. They should be able to immediately recall much, but not necessarily all, of a short story. After a delay, older adults should still recall most of the story but likely not as many details as they do in immediate recall. They should be able to freely recall half of printed words learned but will remember almost all of the words when provided with the item's category (e.g., "the precious stone"). Older adults do well on recognition tasks. They can generate an average of 11 items for a given category within one minute and name a category when provided with specific members. Older adults are slow to complete visual searches, particularly if they have to pay attention to more than one feature of the target, if the distractor letters are similar to the target, or if they do not know where the target is located. They should complete focused-attention and sustained-attention tasks accurately if the target is easily detected. They generally perform slowly on dual-cost tasks (i.e., performing two tasks simultaneously) and have challenges in processing the stimuli, coordinating, and carrying out the responses. Older adults do well on simple, divided-attention tasks but have challenges when tasks are more complex.

The literature also suggests that procedural, prospective, semantic, and remote memory appear to remain intact; however, working memory has considerable age-related declines unless the amount of information is small. Older adults have greater difficulty with the immediate and delayed recall of words, sentences, narrative stories, expository prose, and pictures compared with young and middle-aged adults, and they can forget newly learned information rather quickly. Word-finding problems, particularly recalling names, increase with age. For executive functions, older adults can have poor performance on neuropsychological tests but have preserved reasoning skills needed for real-life situations. Finally, older adults are effective problem solvers who tend to use proactive strategies to solve instrumental problems and passive emotion regulation strategies to deal with interpersonal problems. Neurologically intact adults may be able to do far more than what is reported here, and further research is needed to better document these abilities.

Factors Affecting Older Adults' Cognition and Signs of Problems

Several factors can adversely affect older adults' cognitive abilities. Not surprisingly, deficits in one area of cognition can negatively impact other cognitive abilities. Aging adults' attention and memory can be negatively affected if they are stressed, fatigued, not feeling well, depressed, anxious about a situation or their performance, or taking certain medications (Cohen & Faulkner, 1986; McDougall, Montgomery, Eddy, Jackson, Nelson, & Stark, 2003; Rogers, 2000; Yaffe, Blackwell,

Gore, Sands, Reus, & Browner, 1999). Older adults typically find attention and memory tasks difficult when they demand a great deal of cognitive resources (e.g., complex visual searches, lengthy instructions), they have specific time constraints, they include information that is unfamiliar, or the information is presented in background noise (Craik, 2000; Crawford & Channon, 2002; Kemper et al., 2003; Rogers, 2000). Although alterations in visual and hearing status can lead to reduced performance on cognitive tests (Craik, 2000; Lindenberger & Baltes, 1994), the impact of age-related sensory changes (e.g., vision, hearing, touch, smell) on cognition is not well understood (Schneider & Pichora-Fuller, 1999).

Several signs can indicate that older adults are having cognitive difficulties and should be referred to an SLP or other medical professionals. Overt complaints of not being able to pay attention or remember information should warrant a referral to a physician. Self-reported cognitive problems may be one of the earliest signs of Alzheimer's disease (AD; Crooks, Petitti, Brody, & Yep, 2005; Jonker, Geerlings, & Schmand, 2000). Aging adults who have difficulty ignoring background noise may have impaired attention and memory abilities (see Kemper et al., 2003, for a review), may suffer from a hearing loss, or may have a combination of the two. In such instances, older adults should be seen by their physician, an audiologist, and an SLP. If older adults struggle in carrying out everyday activities, they should be seen by a medical professional. Such difficulties may go undetected by persons in the early stages of dementia in part because they often do not perceive any challenges in performing well-practiced everyday activities and thus underreport any problems (Carlson et al., 1999). If older adults appear to avoid certain activities, they may be experiencing cognitive declines or they may be lacking confidence in their cognitive abilities (West, Welch, & Yassuda, 2000).

Aging adults who evidence any change or decline in memory could be in the early stages of more severe cognitive impairments, such as AD (Collie et al., 2001). Retrospective studies of patients with probable AD have shown that subtle episodic memory difficulties can be detected as many as 20 years prior to the diagnosis (Elias, Beiser, Wolf, Au, White, & D'Agostino, 2000; Masur, Sliwinski, Lipton, Blau, & Crystal, 1994). In contrast, healthy aging adults can have significant variability in memory performance (Davis & Bernstein, 1992; Zacks & Hasher, 2006), and memory problems can be static and unrelated to any kind of neurodegenerative disease (Crook, Bartus, Ferris, Whitehouse, Cohen, & Gershon, 1986; Gron, Bittner, Schmitz, Wunderlich, Tomczark, & Riepe, 2003). Determining cognitive deterioration can require serial administration of valid and reliable neuropsychological tests over an extended period of time (Collie et al., 2001), as declines may not show up during single administrations of tests. For example, many older adults who fall within the normal range of scores on the *Mini-Mental State Examination* (Folstein, Folstein, & McHugh, 1975), a screening measure of attention, verbal memory, language, and constructional praxis, have declines in cognitive functioning (Carlson et al., 1999). Thus, careful evaluation of cognitive abilities is warranted.

Strategies to Help Older Adults' Cognitive Abilities

Several strategies can aid older adults' cognitive abilities. For example, instructions should be short and simple (Craik, 2000), and older adults should be allowed adequate time to complete cognitive activities. Age-related vision and hearing changes should be addressed. Also, aging adults can have better attentional skills if they are familiar with or interested in what is occurring (Rogers, 2000). Thus, using tasks or topics that they find motivating can be helpful. Providing cues and specific practice may facilitate favorable outcomes for divided-attention tasks and dual-task processing but not necessarily on selective attention visual searches (Baron & Mattila, 1989; Fisk & Rogers, 1991; Hartley, 1992; Murphy, Schmitt, Caruso, & Sanders, 1987; Rogers, 2000; Verhaegen, Marcoen, & Goossens, 1992). Memory strategies can also be useful. Episodic memory can be enhanced by including supportive context during the encoding and retrieval stages, such as providing the letters of the target words, offering key words, or giving a descriptive phrase (Craik, 2000; West et al., 2000). Older adults are able to learn complex memory techniques that can lead to beneficial results for several months; however, training must be task specific, and the instructions need to be clearly presented in a step-by-step format (Ericsson, 1985; Ericsson & Kintsch, 1995; West et al., 2000). Combined visual and verbal instructions appear to work best (West et al., 2000), whether done in person or by taking advantage of such technology as DVDs, videos, or possibly podcasts.

Recalling words, particularly names, can be especially challenging for older adults. Several tactics may be useful when recalling names: using circumlocution and synonyms, using mnemonics, mentally running through the alphabet, generating names from a single context (e.g., names of all neighbors), reliving past experiences to enhance the description of the person, and looking up the individual's name (Brooks, Friedman, Gibson, & Yesavage, 1993; Cohen & Faulkner, 1986; Reese, Cherry, & Norris, 1999). Creating a mental image that relates to a specific word or a name can help link the meaning of the word with an interactive image (Brehmer, Li, Straube, Stoll, von Oertzen, Muller, & Lindenberger, 2008; Einstein & McDaniel, 2004; Reese et al., 1999).

Examples include associating the name of "Gordon" with the image of a "garden" (Cohen & Faulkner, 1986) or associating the street name of "Edgemont" with an image of a person standing on the edge of a mountain.

Executive functions and problem solving can be positively impacted. Limiting environmental distractions (e.g., turning off the television) and using compensatory aids, such as timers and color-coded cards to help with sequential activities (e.g., preparing a meal), can help older adults' executive functions (Carlson et al., 1999). Despite potential resistance to such strategies, aging adults will likely be more willing to use them if it means they can continue to maintain their independence (Carlson et al., 1999). With respect to problem-solving skills, ensuring aging adults are involved in situations that require such skills can be beneficial. Similar to that old adage "practice makes perfect," the more older adults succeed in problem solving, the more likely they will continue to be good problem solvers (Crawford & Channon, 2002).

Certain activities can help maintain cognitive functioning and possibly stave off age-related declines. Regular physical exercise is repeatedly recognized in the literature as a way for aging adults to preserve their cognition (Rogers, Meyer, & Mortel, 1990; Scarmeas, Levy, Tang, Manly, & Stern, 2001; Sorond, Schnyer, Serrador, Milberg, & Lipsitz, 2008). Exercise helps maintain cerebral blood flow, which is important because cognitive alterations can in part result from significant age-related changes in the frontal lobes (Sorond et al., 2008). Some authors report that combined strength training and aerobic exercise leads to better cognitive functioning than aerobic exercise alone (Colcombe & Kramer, 2003), although more research is needed to confirm this finding. Being involved in intellectually and socially stimulating leisure activities results in more favorable cognitive functioning (Carlson et al., 1999; Scarmeas & Stern, 2003). Activities such as reading, playing games, taking classes, volunteering, working, being involved in groups (e.g., Sertoma, Red Hat Society), and having social ties with spouses, relatives, and friends can all positively impact older adults' cognition (Balfour, Masaki, White, & Launer, 2001; Scarmeas et al., 2001).

Quick Facts

- General Cognitive Abilities of Neurologically Intact Older Adults:
  - Accurately answer orientation and biographical questions
  - Accurately answer most of the questions pertaining to short stories, and recall the majority of details of a short story immediately after hearing it

- Recall many of the details of a short story following a delay after hearing it, but likely will not include as many details as with immediate recall
- Freely recall approximately half of printed words learned and recall nearly all words when given a category-specific cue (e.g., "the fish")
- Accurately recognize whether or not listed words match ones previously seen
- Generate an average of 11 items for a given category within one minute and name a category when provided with specific members
- Are slow to complete visual searches
- Accurately complete focused attention and sustained attention tasks if the target is easily detected
- Perform dual-cost tasks slowly with challenges in coordinating and carrying out responses
- Accurately complete simple divided-attention tasks but have challenges when tasks are more complex
- Do not have significant changes in procedural, semantic, and remote memory
- Can have considerable age-related declines in working memory unless the amount of information to retain and manipulate is small
- Have difficulty with immediate and delayed recall of words, sentences, narrative stories, expository prose, and pictures compared with young and middle-aged adults
- Forget newly learned information rather quickly
- Demonstrate word-finding problems, particularly when recalling names
- Can have poor executive function performance on neuropsychological tests but have preserved reasoning abilities needed for real-life situations
- Are effective at problem solving; can have fewer but higher-quality solutions
- Use proactive strategies to solve instrumental problems and passive emotion regulation strategies to deal with interpersonal problems
- Factors That Can Negatively Affect Older Adults' Cognition:
  - Not feeling well, taking certain medications, or experiencing stress, fatigue, depression, or anxiety
  - Tasks that demand significant cognitive resources, such as those needed for complex visual searches or those that have lengthy instructions
  - Cognitive tasks that must be completed in a specific period of time

- Target information that is unfamiliar or presented in background noise
- Presence of age-related changes in visual and hearing status that are not addressed
- Signs That an Older Adult Should Be Referred to a Speech-Language Pathologist or Other Medical Professionals:
  - Overt complaints of not being able to pay attention or remember information
  - Difficulty ignoring background noise
  - Struggling to carry out everyday activities or avoiding certain activities
  - Evidence of any memory changes or declines
- Strategies That Can Help Older Adults' Cognition:
  - Attention:
    - Have activities or tasks that are familiar or interesting
    - Keep instructions short and simple
    - Provide cues and task-specific training
  - Memory:
    - Use supportive context during encoding and retrieval stages. For example, provide letters of target words, offer key words, or give descriptive phrases
    - Train memory techniques that are task specific, are clearly stated in a step-by-step format, and combine both verbal and visual instruction
    - Encourage use of circumlocutions and synonyms during word retrieval
    - Encourage use of strategies to recall names. For example, run through the alphabet, generate names from a single context (e.g., naming all neighbors), relive past experiences to enhance the description of the person, look up the name
    - Help the person create a mental image that can be associated with a specific word or name
  - Executive Functions and Problem Solving:
    - Limit environmental distractions (e.g., shut off the television)
    - Use compensatory strategies, such as timers or color-coded cards, for sequential activities (e.g., meal preparation)
    - Encourage active involvement in problem-solving situations
  - In General:
    - Encourage physical exercise
    - Address age-related changes in vision and hearing
    - Encourage the person to participate in intellectually

and socially stimulating leisure activities such as reading, playing games, taking classes, volunteering, working, being involved in groups (e.g., Sertoma, Red Hat Society), and maintaining social ties with spouses, relatives, friends
  ○ Keep instructions short and simple, and allow time to complete activities

Discussion Questions

1. Is there any information that surprised you in terms of what older adults can do or in which they have difficulty?
2. How do depression and anxiety affect attention and memory?
3. How do the older adults in your life show good problem-solving skills, and how do they manage any memory challenges they have?
4. At what point are normal cognitive declines and memory loss considered to be dementia?

References

Baddeley, A. (2003). Working memory: Looking back and looking forward. *Nature Reviews Neuroscience, 4*, 829–839.

Balfour, J. L., Masaki, K., White, L., & Launer, L. J. (2001). The effect of social engagement and productive activity on incident dementia: The Honolulu Asia aging study. *Neurology, 56* (Suppl.), A239.

Baron, A., & Mattila, W. (1989). Response slowing of older adults: Effects of time-limit contingencies on single- and dual-task performances. *Psychology and Aging, 4*, 66–72.

Bayles, K. A., & Tomoeda, C. K. (1993). *Arizona Battery for Communication Disorders of Dementia.* Tucson, AZ: Canyonlands Publishing.

Berardi, A., Parasuraman, R., & Haxby, J. (2001). Overall vigilance and sustained attention decrements in healthy aging. *Experimental Aging Research, 27*, 19–39.

Blanchard-Fields, F., Chen, Y., & Norris, L. (1997). Everyday problem solving across the adult life span: Influence of domain specificity and cognitive appraisal. *Psychology and Aging, 12*, 684–693.

Blanchard-Fields, F., Jahnke, H., & Camp, C. (1995). Age differences in problem-solving style: The role of emotional salience. *Psychology and Aging, 10*, 173–180.

Blanchard-Fields, F., Mienaltowski, A., & Baldi Seay, R. (2007). Age differences in everyday problem-solving effectiveness: Older adults select more effective strategies for interpersonal problems. *Journal of Gerontology: Psychological Sciences, 62B*, P61–P64.

Brehmer, Y., Li, S., Straube, B., Stoll, G., von Oertzen, T., Muller, V., & Lindenberger, U. (2008). Comparing memory skill maintenance across the life span: Preservation in adults, increase in children. *Psychology and Aging, 23*, 227–238.

Brooks, J. O., Friedman, L., Gibson, J. M., & Yesavage, J. A. (1993). Spontaneous mnemonic strategies used by older and younger adults to remember proper names. *Memory, 1*, 393–407.

Brown, J. (1958). Some tests of the decay theory of immediate memory. *Quarterly Journal of Experimental Psychology, 10,* 12–21.

Burda, A. N. (2008). *Healthy aging adults' performance on tests of cognition.* Adele Whitenack Davis Research in Gerontology Award, University of Northern Iowa.

Carlson, M. C., Fried, L. P., Xue, Q. L., Bandeen-Roche, K., Zeger, S. L., & Brandt, J. (1999). Association between executive attention and physical functional performance in community-dwelling older women. *Journal of Gerontology: Social Sciences, 54B,* S262–S270.

Chasteen, A. L., Park, D. C., & Schwartz, N. (2009). Implementation intentions and facilitation of prospective memory. *Psychological Science, 12,* 457–461.

Cohen, G., & Faulkner, D. (1986). Memory for proper names: Age differences in retrieval. *British Journal of Developmental Psychology, 4,* 187–197.

Colcombe, S., & Kramer, A. F. (2003). Fitness effects on the cognitive function of older adults: A meta-analytic study. *Psychological Science, 14,* 125–130.

Collie, A., Maruff, P., Shafiq-Antonacci, R., Smith, M., Hallup, M., Schofield, P. R. et al. (2001). Memory decline in healthy older people: Implications for identifying mild cognitive impairment. *Neurology, 56,* 1533–1538.

Connor, L. T. (2001). Memory in old age: Patterns of decline and perseveration. *Seminars in Speech and Language, 22,* 117–125.

Cornelius, S. W., & Capsi, A. (1987). Everyday problem solving in adulthood and old age. *Psychology and Aging, 2,* 144–153.

Cowan, N. (2001). The magical number 4 in short-term memory: A reconsideration of mental storage capacity. *Behavioral and Brain Science, 24,* 87–185.

Cowan, N. (2008). What are the differences between long-term, short-term, and working memory? *Progress in Brain Research, 169,* 323–338.

Craik, F. I. M. (2000). Age-related changes in human memory. In D. Park & N. Schwarz (Eds.), *Cognitive aging: A primer* (pp. 75–92). Philadelphia: Psychology Press.

Craik, F. I. M., & Jennings, J. M. (1992). Human memory. In F. I. M. Craik & T. A. Salthouse (Eds.), *The handbook of aging and cognition* (pp. 51–110). Hillsdale, NJ: Erlbaum.

Crawford, S., & Channon, S. (2002). Dissociation between performance on abstract tests of executive function and problem solving in real-life type situations in normal aging. *Aging and Mental Health, 6,* 12–21.

Crook, T., Bartus, R. T., Ferris, S. H., Whitehouse, P., Cohen, G. D., & Gershon, S. (1986). Age-associated memory impairment: Proposed diagnostic criteria measures of clinical change. Report of a National Institute of Mental Health Work Group. *Developmental Neuropsychology, 2,* 261–276.

Crooks, V. C., Petitti, D. B., Brody, K. K., & Yep, R. L. (2005). Self-reported severe memory problems as a screen for cognitive impairment and dementia. *Dementia, 4,* 539–551.

Davis, H. P., & Bernstein, P. A. (1992). Age-related changes in explicit and implicit memory. In L. R. Squire & N. Butters (Eds.), *Neuropsychology of memory* (2nd ed.) (pp. 112–124). New York: The Guilford Press.

Davis, H. P., Small, S. A., Stern, Y., Mayeux, R., Feldstein, S. N., & Keller, F. R. (2003). Acquisition, recall, and forgetting of verbal information in long-term memory by young, middle-aged, and elderly individuals. *Cortex, 39,* 1063–1091.

Dobbs, A. R., & Rule, B. G. (1989). Adult age differences in working memory. *Psychology and Aging, 4,* 500–503.

Duckworth, M., Iezzi, T., & O'Donohue, W. (2008). *Motor vehicle collisions: Medical, psychosocial, and legal consequences.* Boston, MA: Elsevier Academic.

Einstein, G. O., & McDaniel, M. A. (2004). *Memory fitness: A guide for successful aging.* New Haven, CT: Yale University Press.

Elias, M. F., Beiser, A., Wolf, P. A., Au, R., White, R. F., & D'Agostino, R. B. (2000). The preclinical phase of Alzheimer's disease: A 22-year prospective study of the Framingham cohort. *Archives of Neurology, 57,* 808–813.

Enns, J. T., & Trick, L. M. (2006). Four modes of selection. In E. Bialystok & F. I. M. Craik (Eds.), *Lifespan cognition: Mechanisms of change* (pp. 43–56). New York: Oxford University Press.

Ericsson, K. A. (1985). Memory skill. *Canadian Journal of Psychology, 39,* 188–231.

Ericsson, K. A., & Kintsch, W. (1995). Long term working memory. *Psychological Review, 102,* 211–245.

Fisk, A. D., & Rogers, W. (1991). Toward an understanding of age-related memory and visual search effects. *Journal of Experimental Psychology: General, 120,* 131–149.

Folstein, M. F., Folstein, S. E., & McHugh, P. R. (1975). Mini-Mental State: A practical method for grading the cognitive state of patients for the clinician. *Journal of Psychiatric Research, 12,* 189–198.

Giambra, L. M. (1993). Sustained attention in older adults: Performance and processes. In J. Cerella, J. Rybash, W. Hoyer, & M. L. Commons (Eds.), *Adult information processing: Limits on loss* (pp. 259–272). San Diego, CA: Academic Press.

Gron, G., Bittner, D., Schmitz, B., Wunderlich, A. P., Tomczark, R., & Riepe, M. W. (2003). Variability in memory performance in aged healthy individuals: An fMRI study. *Neurobiology of Aging, 24,* 453–463.

Hartley, A. (1992). Attention. In F. I. M. Craik & T. Salthouse (Eds.), *Handbook of aging and cognition* (pp. 3–49). Hillsdale, NJ: Erlbaum.

Hedden, T., & Gabrieli, D. E. (2004). Insights into the aging mind: A view from cognitive neuroscience. *Nature Reviews Neuroscience, 5,* 87–96.

Helm-Estabrooks, N. (2001). *Cognitive Linguistic Quick Test.* San Antonio, TX: The Psychological Corporation.

Hultsch, D. R., & Dixon, R. A. (1984). Memory for text materials in adulthood. In P. B. Baltes & O. G. Brim (Eds.), *Life-span development and behavior,* vol. 6. New York: Academic Press.

James, L. (2006). Specific effects of aging on proper name retrieval: Now you see them, now you don't. *Journal of Gerontology, 61B,* 180–183.

Jenkins, L., Myerson, J., Hale, S., & Fry, A. (1999). Individual and developmental differences in working memory across the life span. *Psychonomic Bulletin & Review, 6,* 28–40.

Jonker, C., Geerlings, M. I., & Schmand, B. (2000). Are memory complaints predictive for dementia? A review of clinical and population-based studies. *International Journal of Geriatric Psychiatry, 15,* 983–991.

Kemper, S. (1987). Syntactic complexity and elderly adults' prose recall. *Experimental Aging Research, 13,* 47–52.

Kemper, S., Herman, R. E., & Lian, C. H. (2003). The costs of doing two things at once for young and older adults: Talking while walking, finger tapping, and ignoring speech or noise. *Psychology and Aging, 18,* 181–192.

Kemper, S., & Sumner, A. (2001). The structure of verbal abilities in young and older adults. *Psychology and Aging, 16,* 312–322.

Kennedy, M., & Coelho, C. (2005). Self-regulation after traumatic brain injury: A framework for intervention of memory and problem solving. *Seminars in Speech and Language, 26,* 242–255.

Kramer, A. F., Humphrey, D. G., Larish, J. F., Logan, G. D., & Strayer, D. L. (1994). Aging and inhibition: Beyond a unitary view of inhibitory processing attention. *Psychology and Aging, 9*, 491–512.

Kramer, A. F., & Kray, J. (2006). Aging and attention. In E. Bialystok & F. I. M. Craik (Eds.), *Lifespan cognition: Mechanisms of change* (pp. 57–69). New York: Oxford University Press.

Light, L. L. (1992). The organization of memory in old age. In F. I. M. Craik & T. A. Salthouse (Eds.), *The handbook of aging and cognition* (pp. 111–165). Hillsdale, NJ: Erlbaum.

Light, L. L., & Burke, D. M. (1988). Patterns of language and memory in old age. In L. L. Light & D. M. Burke (Eds.), *Language, memory, and aging* (pp. 244–271). New York: Cambridge University Press.

Lindenberger, U., & Baltes, P. B. (1994). Sensory functioning and intelligence in old age: A strong connection. *Psychology and Aging, 9*, 339–355.

Masur, D. M., Sliwinski, M., Lipton, R. B., Blau, A. D., & Crystal, H. A. (1994). Neuropsychological prediction of dementia and the absence of dementia in healthy older persons. *Neurology, 44*, 1427–1432.

McDougall, G. J., Montgomery, K. S., Eddy, N., Jackson, E., Nelson, E., & Stark, T. (2003). Aging memory self-efficacy: Elders share their thoughts and experiences. *Geriatric Nursing, 24*, 162–168.

Miller, G. A. (1956). The magical number seven, plus or minus two: Some limits of our capacity for processing information. *Psychological Review, 63*, 81–97.

Murphy, M., Schmitt, F., Caruso, M., & Sanders, R. (1987). Metamemory in older adults: The role of monitoring in serial recall. *Psychology and Aging, 2*, 331–339.

Naveh-Benjamin, M., Hussain, Z., Guez, J., & Bar-On, M. (2003). Adult age differences in episodic memory: Further support for an associative-deficit hypothesis. *Journal of Experimental Psychology: Learning, Memory, and Cognition, 29*, 826–837.

Park, D. C., & Payer, D. (2006). Working memory across the adult lifespan. In E. Bialystok & F. I. M. Craik (Eds.), *Lifespan cognition: Mechanisms of change* (pp. 128–142). New York: Oxford University Press.

Peterson, L. R., & Peterson, M. J. (1959). Short-term retention of individual items. *Journal of Experimental Psychology, 58*, 193–198.

Phillips, L. H., & Della Salla, S. (1998). Aging, intelligence, and anatomical segregation in the frontal lobes. *Learning and Individual Differences, 10*, 217–243.

Plude, D. J., & Doussard-Roosevelt, J. A. (1989). Aging, selective attention, and feature integration. *Psychology and Aging, 4*, 98–105.

Posner, M. (2008). Attention as a cognitive and neural system. *Current Directions in Psychological Science, 1*, 11.

Reese, C. M., Cherry, K. E., & Norris, L. E. (1999). Practical memory concerns for older adults. *Journal of Clinical Geropsychology, 5*, 231–244.

Rey, A. (1964). *L'Examin clinique en psychologie*. Paris: Press Universitaires de France.

Riddle, D. (2007). *Brain aging: Models, methods, and mechanisms*. Boca Raton, FL: CRC Press.

Rogers, R. L., Meyer, J. S., & Mortel, K. F. (1990). After reaching retirement age, physical activity sustains cerebral perfusion and cognition. *Journal of the American Geriatrics Society, 38*, 123–128.

Rogers, W. A. (2000). Attention and aging. In D. Park & N. Schwarz (Eds.), *Cognitive aging: A primer* (pp. 57–73). Philadelphia: Psychology Press.

Ross-Swain, D. (1996). *Ross Information Processing Assessment* (2nd ed.). Austin, TX: Pro-Ed.

Ross-Swain, D., & Fogle, P. T. (1996). *Ross Information Processing Assessment–Geriatric*. Austin, TX: Pro-Ed.

Salthouse, T. (2000). Aging and measures of processing speed. *Biological Psychology, 54,* 35–54.

Salthouse, T. A. (1982). *Adult cognition: An experimental psychology of human aging*. New York: Springer-Verlag.

Salthouse, T. A. (1991). *Theoretical perspectives on cognitive aging*. Hillsdale, NJ: Erlbaum.

Scarmeas, N., Levy, G., Tang, M., Manly, J., & Stern, Y. (2001). Influence of leisure activity on the incidence of Alzheimer's disease. *Neurology, 57,* 2236–2242.

Scarmeas, N., & Stern, Y. (2003). Cognitive reserve and lifestyle. *Journal of Clinical and Experimental Neuropsychology, 25,* 625–633.

Schneider, B. A., & Pichora-Fuller, M. K. (1999). Implications of perceptual deterioration for cognitive aging research. In F. I. M. Craik & T. A. Salthouse (Eds.), *The handbook of aging and cognition* (2nd ed.) (pp. 155–219). Mahwah, NJ: Erlbaum.

Simpson, G. B., Kellas, G., & Ferraro, F. R. (1999). Age and the allocation of attention across the time course of word recognition. *Journal of General Psychology, 126,* 119–136.

Sorond, F. A., Schnyer, D. M., Serrador, J. M., Milberg, W. P., & Lipsitz, L. A. (2008). Cerebral blood flow regulation during cognitive tasks: Effects on healthy aging. *Cortex, 44,* 179–184.

Verghese, J., Buschke, H., Viola, L., Hall, C., Kuslansky, G., & Lipton, R. (2002). Validity of divided attention tasks in predicting falls in older individuals: A preliminary study. *Journal of the American Geriatrics Society, 50,* 1572–1576.

Verhaegen, P., Marcoen, A., & Goossens, L. (1992). Improving memory performance in the aged through mnemonic training: A meta-analytic study. *Psychology and Aging, 7,* 242–251.

West, R. L., Welch, D. C., & Yassuda, M. S. (2000). Innovative approaches to memory training for older adults. In R. D. Hill, L. Bäckman, & A. Stigsdotter Neely (Eds.), *Cognitive rehabilitation in old age* (pp. 81–105). New York: Oxford University Press.

Wierenga, C., Benjamin, M., Gopinath, K., Perlstein, W., Leonard, C., Gonzalez Rothi, et al. (2006). Age-related changes in word retrieval: Role of bilateral frontal and subcortical networks. *Neurobiology of Aging, 29,* 197–458.

Yaffe, K., Blackwell, T., Gore, R., Sands, L., Reus, V., & Browner, W. S. (1999). Depressive symptoms and cognitive decline in nondemented older women. *Archives of General Psychiatry, 56,* 425–430.

Zacks, R. T., & Hasher, L. (2006). Aging and long-term memory: Deficits are not inevitable. In E. Bialystok & F. I. M. Craik (Eds.), *Lifespan cognition: Mechanisms of change* (pp. 162–177). New York: Oxford University Press.

Zacks, R. T., Hasher, L., & Li, K. Z. H. (1999). Human memory. In F. I. M. Craik & T. A. Salthouse (Eds.), *The handbook of aging and cognition* (2nd ed.) (pg. 293–358). Mahwah, NJ: Erlbaum.

Chapter 3

Auditory Comprehension

Angela N. Burda, PhD, CCC-SLP

Introduction

We hear and process an enormous amount of auditory input every day. Our ability to make sense of what we hear helps us determine whether or not it is the alarm clock going off in the early hours of the morning or the ringing of a phone. We can differentiate between the timer on the oven and the siren of a fire truck. We are also able to comprehend what other people say, which in turn, allows us to be able to respond to them appropriately. While our comprehension of speech can seem nearly effortless, it is actually a very complex process. Making sense out of a message requires rapid identification and processing of individual speech sounds and words, then integrating other incoming words and sentences with what was previously spoken or stored (Pichora-Fuller, Schneider, & Daneman, 1995; Thornton & Light, 2006). Readers are able to go back and reread a message in front of them, but listeners do not have that luxury. Asking speakers to repeat what they said may not be an option. As a result, some listeners have more trouble trying to determine what they are hearing.

Not surprisingly, aspects of cognition, such as memory, can factor heavily into the understanding of speech (Caplan & Waters, 1999; see Chapter 2 on cognition). Auditory processing is challenging for listeners who are unable to attend to or remember what was said. Various theoretical perspectives address age-related changes in comprehension abilities (see Chapter 1 on theoretical perspectives). As with any of the abilities discussed in this book, auditory comprehension can easily be taken for granted. We tend not to think about our auditory processing abilities until difficulties occur. Nonverbal communication is obviously very important when we interact with others. Body language and gestures can help us make sense out of a spoken message; however, the understanding of speech is the cornerstone of our ability to communicate.

This chapter will discuss what aging adults' auditory processing abilities generally should be, factors that can negatively affect older adults' auditory comprehension, signs that may warrant referral to a speech-language pathologist or other medical professionals, and what strategies can help aging adults' auditory comprehension. A list of "Quick Facts" at the end of the chapter summarizes important points. For the purposes of this chapter, the terms *auditory comprehension, auditory processing, speech understanding,* and *speech perception* are used interchangeably.

Older Adults' General Auditory Comprehension Abilities

Speech-language pathologists (SLPs) who work with adults must evaluate their patients' language comprehension and expression. Assessment tools divide these broad language areas into subtests (e.g., Auditory Comprehension, Writing) and in many cases arrange items hierarchically. Thus, subtests begin with directions and/or responses that are shorter and simpler in nature and progress to lengthier, more complex items (Bayles & Tomoeda, 1993; Helm-Estabrooks, 1992; Keenan & Brassell, 1975). In several of the commercially available language tests for adults, auditory-comprehension tasks generally involve following commands of increasing complexity and answering questions of increasing difficulty. Questions can be related to personal information, to general knowledge of the world, or to stories that individuals hear read aloud by the SLP (Bayles & Tomoeda, 1993; Goodglass, Kaplan, & Barresi, 2001; Helm-Estabrooks, 1992; Kertesz, 2006).

Finding information about neurologically intact aging adults' auditory comprehension abilities can be challenging. Research studies have not necessarily evaluated clinical tasks found in speech-language pathology tests, such as those previously mentioned (e.g., commands of increasing length). Tests do not systematically include aging adults as part of the standardization process, nor do they specify the ages of the normal adults in the assessment manuals. In certain cases, the normal group could be considered questionable. For example, the *Aphasia Language Performance Scale* (ALPS; Keenan & Brassell, 1975) used only prisoners in the group of normal adults for its standardization sample. The authors reported that they wanted participants who roughly estimated the abilities of Veterans Administration patients, which in their opinion, included persons who were neither highly educated nor intelligent. Although including adults who represent a variety of socioeconomic status and intellectual levels would be helpful as part of a test standardization, incarcerated individuals do not provide a good example of normal language performance, as many individuals in the penal system have language disorders (Blanton & Degenais, 2007). When tests have included normal aging adults, these individuals have not necessarily been a separate control group. Some exceptions exist, and information found in test manuals, coupled with empirical data in the literature, can provide a general guide of what the expected auditory comprehension abilities are for neurologically intact older adults.

The *Aphasia Diagnostic Profile* (ADP; Helm-Estabrooks, 1992) is one test in which older adults participated in the standardization process. Data from 40 neurologically intact adults aged 20–99 years were included. Although 11 of these adults fell within the age range of 60–99, the test's author did not report the normative data by specific age groups. The Auditory Language Comprehension section of the ADP includes: Following Commands (e.g., "Close your eyes," "Where is your heart?"); Comprehension of Single Words, in which patients identify a picture in a field of four black-and-white line drawings; and Understanding Stories, in which individuals answer yes/no questions after listening to three stories of increasing length and complexity. Only one overall score is obtained for Auditory Language Comprehension, meaning that scores are not separated based on the different sections (e.g., Following Commands, Understanding Stories). The total number correct possible for this section is 28 points. The ADP's test manual reports that neurologically intact adults had a mean score of 24.7 (SD = 3.5) out of a possible 28, which is an approximate average of 88% for the combined items in this section. When looking at the data, however, one must keep in mind that the normative sample included adults whose ages ranged from 20 to 99.

The *Arizona Battery for Communication Disorders of Dementia* (ABCD; Bayles & Tomoeda, 1993) is another test that included neurologically intact older adults as part of the standardization process. In fact, it is one of the few tests in which older adults were a separate control group as part of the normative research. The mean age of these individuals was 70.44 years (SD = 17.07). Subtests that assess auditory comprehension include: Following Commands, Comparative Questions, and Story Retelling–Immediate. A Story Retelling–Delayed subtest is part of the test and could be viewed as an auditory-comprehension task, but because the delayed story retelling requires patients to hold information in their short-term memory, it could also be considered a cognitive task. For the Following Commands subtest, directions range from one step (e.g., "Look up"), to two steps (e.g., "Clap, then point"), and up to three steps (e.g., "Cough, smile, then whistle"). Older adults received a mean score of 8.8 items correct ($SD = 0.4$) out of a total of 9 possible, or 98% correct. For the Comparative Questions subtest, participants answer abstract yes/no questions based on general knowledge, such as "Is ice colder than steam?" and "Is a yard longer than a foot?" The neurologically intact older adults achieved a mean of 5.9 ($SD = 0.5$) questions correct out of a total of 6 items possible, or 98% correct. Average scores for these two subtests do not differ significantly from those of a control group of healthy young adults who were included as part of the standardization sample.

As the names of the ABCD's Story Retelling subtests imply, patients are asked to retell a story both immediately after hearing it and then after a delay. The immediate retelling subtest occurs early on in the test, and the delayed retelling is the last task of the entire test. Fifteen subtests are administered between the two story-retelling subtests. No questions pertaining to the story are asked, and patients are prompted at the end of the Story Retelling–Immediate subtest to remember the information because they will be asked about it later. The story is about a woman who was shopping and lost her wallet without realizing it. She later receives a call from a little girl who found the lost wallet. Patients are scored on their ability to report correct information units (e.g., "lady," "her wallet," "phone rang").

Bayles and Tomoeda (1993) report that for the Story Retelling–Immediate subtest, older adults in the normative sample were able to recall an average of 14 information units ($SD = 2.8$) out of a total of 17 information units possible, or 82% correct. On the Story Retelling–Delayed subtest, the older adults recalled an average of 12.4 information units ($SD = 4.5$), which is 73% correct. Scores for the Story Retelling–Immediate subtest do not differ significantly between neurologically intact young and old adults. Performance does, however, differ between the two age groups on the Story Retelling–Delayed subtest; older adults recalled an average of approximately 12 informational units, while young adults recalled nearly 15 informational units. Overall, according to the ABCD, older adults should be able to accurately follow commands of increasing length (up to three steps) and answer abstract yes/no questions pertaining to general knowledge. They should also be able to immediately recall much, but not necessarily all, of a short story. After a delay, older adults should still be able to recall most of the story but will likely have difficulty recalling as many details as they can in the immediate recall.

In addition to collecting information from standardized tests, research studies have focused on older adults' auditory comprehension abilities. Findings from these investigations indicate that older adults can exhibit auditory processing delays when listening to sentences (Federmeier & Kutas, 2005) and narratives (Little, Prentice, Darrow, & Wingfield, 2005). Although processing delays may occur, the good news is that older adults can follow spoken directions (Schmitt & Moore, 1989), understand passages spoken at a normal conversational rate (Schmitt & Moore, 1989), and maintain and possibly even add to their store of vocabulary and word-related knowledge (Salthouse, 1993). Older adults' organization of word knowledge appears to remain fairly stable (Federmeier & Kutas, 2005), allowing them to identify words accurately (Wingfield, Alexander, & Cavigelli, 1994) and draw inferences (Light, Valencia-Laver, & Davis, 1991; Soederberg Miller, Stine-Morrow, Kirkorian, & Conroy, 2004). Thus, if a conversation is related to pets, older adults would be able to access their organizational store of what types of animals are typically kept as pets. If the conversation involved the word *pot-bellied*, the older adult could infer that their communication partner is talking about a pet pig versus a pet cat or dog.

In a study conducted by Burda (2007), 31 adults aged 65 and older were divided into three age categories: Young-Old (ages 65–74; M_{age} = 69.3 years, SD = 2.2), Middle-Old (ages 75–84; M_{age} = 81.1 years, SD = 1.9), and Old-Old (ages 85+; M_{age} = 89.5 years, SD = 4.4). Participants were divided into roughly equal age groups (i.e., 10 participants in Young-Old and Old-Old groups, 11 in Middle-Old group) and were asked to complete a variety of auditory-comprehension tasks that could be clinically evaluated by SLPs. These tasks included having participants follow one-step directions (e.g., "Scratch your head") and complex directions (e.g., "When I snap my fingers, look at the floor"), answer personal yes/no questions (e.g., "Are you a man?"), answer complex yes/no questions related to general world knowledge (e.g., "Do you pay for items that are free of charge?"), and answer wh-questions after hearing two short stories. One story, nine sentences in length, was about baking an apple pie. The other story, seven sentences in length, was about a family's morning routine. Results of this study are included in **Table 3-1**, broken down by age groups.

As shown in Table 3-1, participants had high accuracy levels for the directions and answering personal and complex yes/no questions. Performance was reduced when participants were asked to answer questions after hearing short stories. No marked differences occurred across the age groups, and in some cases, those in the Old-Old group had higher mean scores than participants in the two younger age groups. In addition, no statistically significant differences occurred in performance among the three age groups. It should be noted that the sample size for this pilot study was small.

Table 3-1										
Mean Performance for Auditory-Comprehension Tasks										
		Young-Old			Middle-Old			Old-Old		
Task	Total*	M	SD	%**	M	SD	%**	M	SD	%**
One-step directions	10	10.0	0.0	100	10.0	0.0	100	10.0	0.0	100
Complex directions	10	9.9	0.3	99	9.6	0.7	96	9.6	0.7	96
Personal yes/no Qs	10	10.0	0.0	100	10.0	0.0	100	10.0	0.0	100
Complex yes/no Qs	10	10.0	0.0	100	9.7	0.6	97	9.9	0.3	99
Short story (pie)	10	7.0	2.9	70	6.6	2.4	66	7.4	2.1	74
Short story (morning)	10	7.4	1.7	74	7.7	1.3	77	8.0	1.7	80

Note: *refers to the total number of points possible. **refers to the percentage correct.
Source: Burda (2007).

In summary, based on information included in the normative data for adult language tests and in research studies, older adults should be able to understand and follow directions, identify pictures in a field of four, and answer yes/no questions related to personal information and general world knowledge. Although they should be able to answer many of the yes/no questions pertaining to short stories and be able to immediately recall the important details of a story, their performance on these tasks will likely be lower compared with their performance on the previously mentioned tasks (e.g., following directions). It is possible they may accurately answer only three-fourths of the questions after listening to short stories. During delayed story recall, older adults are expected to include fewer details than in immediate story recall, yet they should still be able to retell most of what they heard. Older adults can exhibit speech processing delays; however, their accumulated vocabulary and word-related knowledge helps them understand the meaning of the speaker's message. It is important to bear in mind that neurologically intact adults may be able to do far more than is reported here since this information is based on a limited amount of available data. More research is needed to better document the abilities of older adults.

Factors Affecting Older Adults' Auditory Comprehension and Signs of Problems

Several factors can make it more difficult for older adults to understand speech. These factors may relate to the speakers, to the environment, or to the aging adults themselves. One factor that pertains to the aged population is that the majority of older adults have some type of hearing loss (Gordon-Salant, 2005). Hearing impairments in the aged can have various causes, including exposure to noise, otologic disease, and oto-toxicity (Dugan, 2003; Lipsky & King, 2005). Many older adults also develop presbycusis, an age-related hearing loss (Corso, 1963; Willott, 1991; Yost, 2007), which generally makes it more difficult to hear high-frequency sounds (van Rooij & Plomp, 1990), such as fricatives (e.g., /sh/, /s/) and affricates (e.g., /ch/), and higher-pitched voices, such as females' and children's voices. Although age-related hearing de-clines can begin in middle age or even earlier, significant changes in hearing may not show up for several years (Mehrotra & Wagner, 2008). These small decrements can still negatively impact speech compre-hension (Thornton & Light, 2006). Although hearing aids can help with speech understanding, not all individuals with a hearing loss opt to use amplification (Garstecki & Erler, 1997; Gordon-Salant, 2005).

Issues related to the environment or the context of the commu-nicative interaction influence older adults' speech perception. For ex-ample, reverberation and background noise can be very problematic. Reverberation is "the prolongation of sound in an enclosed room" (Gordon-Salant, 2005, p. 21) and can be particularly significant in rooms that have high ceilings and walls made of glass, including windows and mirrors (Gordon-Salant, 2005). Older adults, with and without hearing loss, cannot understand speech as accurately as young adults when re-verberation is present (Gordon-Salant & Fitzgibbons, 1993; Helfer & Wilber, 1990; Nabelek & Robinson, 1982).

With respect to background noise, older adults who do not have any hearing loss can still experience greater difficulty understanding speech in noise than younger adults (Gordon-Salant & Fitzgibbons, 1995, 1999). When older adults with presbycusis try to understand speech in background noise, their difficulties only heighten, and they need more time to process what is said (Gordon-Salant & Fitzgibbons, 1995, 1999). In general, difficult listening situations (e.g., presence of background noise, more than one person speaking simultaneously) increase the likelihood that older adults will have problems under-standing what others say (Humes, 1996; Schneider, Daneman, Murphy, & Kwong-See, 2000). Older adults are aware of their difficulties in such conditions and, not surprisingly, report their own challenges in understanding speech when noise is present (see CHABA, 1998, for a review). Unfortunately, noise is often present in daily life, from some-times unexpected sources. The sound of an air conditioner or a softly buzzing light can interfere with aging adults' auditory comprehen-sion in an otherwise quiet situation.

As previously indicated, context plays a significant role in speech comprehension. Aging adults can have greater difficulty understand-ing speech when they do not know the context (Schneider, Daneman, & Murphy, 2005). When the context is highly predictable, older adults are able to accurately indicate what they think the speaker has said (Balota & Duchek, 1991; Burke & Harrold, 1993). If, however, the context does not allow older listeners to predict what the speaker says, they are not as accurate in understanding speech (Dubno, Ahlstrom, & Horwitz, 2000). For example, research studies have found that older adults tend to do much better at accurately repeating the last word in a sentence such as "I've got a cold and a sore *throat*" versus "He is considering the *throat*" because the latter sentence lacks helpful context (Dubno, Ahlstrom, & Horwitz, 2000).

Speakers also influence the degree to which aging adults understand what is said. Older adults have greater difficulty understanding speech when they are not familiar with an individual's speaking pattern (Yonan & Sommers, 2000) or if speech is altered in some manner. For example, a fast speech rate can negatively affect aging adults' speech comprehension (Gordon-Salant & Fitzgibbons, 1995, 1999; Tun, 1998). The rate of normal conversational speech reportedly ranges from 175 to 275 words per minute (Schmitt & Moore, 1989; Wingfield, Poon, Lombardi, & Lowe, 1985; Yorkston & Beukelman, 1984). However, when persons use faster speaking rates, older adults can have delayed or inaccurate processing, even if a single phrase of a sentence is spoken too rapidly (Gordon-Salant & Fitzgibbons, 2004). Consonants in particular can be hard for aging adults to process because the acoustic information is so brief (Gordon-Salant, 2005). The presence of a speaker's foreign accent can also make accurate speech perception difficult for aging adults (Burda, Bradley-Potter, Dralle, Murphy, & Roehs, 2009; Burda, Casey, Foster, Pilkington, & Reppe, 2006; Burda & Hageman, 2005; Burda, Scherz, Hageman, & Edwards, 2003). Much like rapid speech, accented speech is not considered disordered (ASHA, 2007). However, non-native English speakers can have articulatory, prosodic, and grammatical differences that make it more difficult for listeners to understand what they are saying (Clarke, 2002; Edwards & Strattman, 1996; Major, Fitzmaurice, Bunta, & Balasubramanian, 2002; Munro & Derwing, 1995a, 1995b).

Auditory processing can require more effort for older adults if any of these factors are present (hearing loss, fast speaking rate, unknown context, etc.), leaving them to depend more on top-down processing. Top-down processing means that listeners have to rely on their own knowledge of the world to help them make sense out of what they are hearing. For example, if an elderly individual sees that the neighbor children are throwing a ball back and forth, the aging adult has the general knowledge that "children play." The older adult might ask the children what they are doing. Even before they answer, the older neighbor can presuppose that the children are involved in some sort of game or activity that they find enjoyable and would refer to as "playing." Thus, if the children take time to describe in detail the rules and other particulars of their game, the older adult can focus his or her efforts into understanding these details because he or she understands the overarching concept of "kids playing." The challenge is that when older adults need to rely more on top-down processing, they have less effort available to focus on what the speaker is saying, possibly missing valuable information.

Several signs can indicate older adults are having difficulty with auditory comprehension and/or hearing and should be referred to a speech-language pathologist or other medical professionals. Obviously, overt complaints of not being able to hear or understand speech would warrant a referral to an audiologist. Many aging adults do not want to be obvious in their challenges understanding speech and will instead exhibit more covert signs, such as difficulty following or participating in a conversation; problems carrying out activities after hearing the directions; asking for frequent clarifications of what was said; having inappropriate responses, topic shifts, and turn-taking during a communicative interaction; or sticking to topics that are superficial in nature (Tye-Murray, 2004). Older adults who have difficulty understanding speech may also withdraw from social activities and other endeavors that they previously enjoyed (Tye-Murray, 2004). However, reasons other than declines in auditory comprehension and hearing can lead to the same types of behaviors. For example, depression can cause people to withdraw socially (Markowitz, 2008). Early signs of dementia can lead to inappropriate responses during conversation (Powell, Hale, & Bayer, 1995; Santo Pietro & Ostuni, 2003). Regardless, if these signs occur, older individuals would benefit from being seen by the appropriate medical professionals.

Strategies to Help Older Adults' Auditory Comprehension

Several strategies can enhance the auditory comprehension of older adults. Ensuring that the environment is as quiet as possible is helpful. Aging adults with normal hearing can generally understand speech in ideal, quiet listening conditions (Gordon-Salant & Fitzgibbons, 1999; Pichora-Fuller, Schneider, & Daneman, 1995). A quiet environment alone will not necessarily make understanding speech easy for them. Many older adults with no significant hearing loss and normal speech reception thresholds report that understanding speech is frequently tiring or takes a great deal of effort (Pichora-Fuller, Schneider, & Daneman, 1995; Schneider, Daneman, Pichora-Fuller, 2002). Despite the increased effort, however, these individuals can comprehend what speakers are saying. Older adults can improve their speech perception if they are fitted for and wear hearing aids (Garstecki & Erler, 1997) or use assistive listening devices (Gordon-Salant, 2005). For those who already have hearing aids or other amplification devices, making sure that these devices are working properly and that the batteries are not dead, are necessities. Some communication partners will speak very loudly when talking to older adults who have a hearing loss. This can be a fine line; although older adults may benefit from increased volume to some degree, if speech is too loud, most listeners are unable to adequately understand what is being said (Martin & Greer Clark, 2006). Therefore, it is helpful for the speaker to ask older adults whether they are speaking loud enough or too loudly.

The use of prosody when speaking allows older adults to reduce their processing demands and better decode what is being said (Cohen & Faulkner, 1986; Kjelgaard, Titone, & Wingfield, 1999; Wingfield, Lahar, & Stine, 1989; Wingfield, Lindfield, & Goodglass, 2000; Wingfield, Wayland, & Stine, 1992). Prosody provides the melodic contour and rhythm of speech (Meyers, 1999; Wennerstrom, 2001), and it allows older listeners to determine which syllables are stressed and how many syllables are being spoken (Wingfield, Lindfield, & Goodglass, 2000). In addition, aging adults can determine if the speaker is asking a question or making a statement based on the intonation pattern. They can also pick up on the particular words that are stressed to get a general idea of the topic. Thus, speakers should incorporate natural-sounding prosody into their speech, as auditory comprehension problems can arise when speakers have a flat intonation pattern or when many widely ranging intonation changes occur (Edwards & Strattman, 1996).

Familiarity can also aid older adults' speech comprehension. As previously mentioned, when older adults know the context of what is being said, they can better understand speech (Dubno, Ahlstrom, & Horwitz, 2000; Federmeier & Kutas, 2005; Pichora-Fuller, Schneider, & Daneman, 1995). Thus, having some degree of familiarity with the topic can be helpful. The caveat is that listeners tend to benefit the most when they learn of the topic beforehand versus after the fact (Wingfield, Alexander, & Cavigelli, 1994). This is not surprising. If we happen upon a group of people who invite us to join them in the conversation but neglect to tell us what they are talking about, we can spend a great deal of time just trying to figure out the topic. It would be helpful for someone to say "We're talking about last night's football game." Even more helpful would be if this information was offered before the conversation picked up again, instead of when it was over. In sum, older adults can benefit from a type of "heads-up" about what they are going to hear.

Context also helps older adults disambiguate word meanings (Federmeier, 2006). For example, homonyms (also referred to as homophones) are words that sound the same but have different spellings and different meanings. *See* and *sea* are homonyms, and knowing the context lets older adults accurately discern which of these words the speaker is using. Another way to add familiarity to a spoken message is to build in repetition and redundancy (Pichora-Fuller, 2008). Speakers can facilitate comprehension by repeating, rephrasing, or summarizing what they have said.

Older adults' auditory comprehension can also improve when they become familiar with an individual's manner of speaking (Gass & Varonis, 1984; Yonan & Sommers, 2000), including non-native English speakers who have an accent (Burda, Overhake, & Thompson, 2005). Being accustomed to speakers' voices can even improve speech understanding in noisy listening situations (Yonan & Sommers, 2000). Listeners can become familiar with an individual's speaking manner when they have more than one opportunity to hear the speaker. Even when this is not possible, older adults can still become more familiar with specific speech patterns over the course of a single listening session (Burda et al., 2005).

Since a great deal of research indicates fast speech can cause difficulty for older adults (Gordon-Salant & Fitzgibbons, 1995, 1999; Tun, 1998), speakers should take care to speak at an appropriate rate; however, speaking at a much slower than normal rate is not necessarily helpful (Kemper & Harden, 1999; Nejime & Moore, 1998). Similar to speech that is too loud, speech that is too slow can be difficult for older adults to understand. In addition to using appropriate speaking rates to aid auditory processing, older adults may need more time to process what is being said. Studies have shown that older adults take more pause time at "wrap-up" points in phrases and sentences, and that these pauses help auditory processing (Little, Prentice, Darrow, & Wingfield, 2005). Thus, allowing adequate processing time can lead to better speech comprehension.

Quick Facts

- General Auditory Comprehension Abilities of Neurologically Intact Older Adults:
  - Understand and follow directions that range from simple to multistep
  - Demonstrate comprehension of single words by identifying a picture in a field of four
  - Answer yes/no questions related to personal information and general world knowledge
  - Answer most of the questions pertaining to short stories, and recall the majority of details of a short story immediately after hearing it
  - Recall many of the details of a short story following a delay after hearing it, but likely will not include as many details as with immediate recall

- Can have speech-processing delays
- Maintain and possibly even strengthen vocabulary and word-related knowledge
- Factors That Can Negatively Affect Older Adults' Auditory Comprehension:
  - Presence of a hearing loss, including presbycusis, an age-related hearing loss
  - Presence of background noise or more than one person speaking at a time
  - Lack of context of what is being said
  - Speakers who use a fast rate, have an accent, or speak in a manner that is unfamiliar to the older listener
- Signs That an Older Adult Should Be Referred to a Speech-Language Pathologist or Other Medical Professionals:
  - Overt complaints of not being able to hear or understand speech
  - Covert signs of not being able to hear or understand speech, including:
    - Difficulty following or participating in a conversation
    - Problems carrying out activities after hearing the directions
    - Asking for frequent clarifications of what was said
    - Having inappropriate responses, topic shifts, and turn-taking during a conversation
    - Sticking to topics that are superficial in nature
  - Withdrawing from social activities or other activities previously enjoyed

(Note: If compromised hearing is suspected, refer individual to an audiologist.)

- Strategies That Can Help Older Adults' Auditory Comprehension:
  - Provide a quiet listening environment
  - Manage any hearing loss. If hearing aids are worn or assistive listening devices are used, ensure they are in working order and that the batteries are not dead
  - Speak at a volume level that is comfortable for the older listener and allows the person to understand what is being said; do not speak too loudly
  - Speak at a rate at which older adults can understand speech; do not speak too fast or too slow
  - Speak with prosodic variation, using natural changes in intonation and stress patterns
  - Tell older adults what the topic of the conversation is going to be or give them a "heads up" about what they are going to hear

- Allow older listeners to become familiar with the way a person speaks. Repeated exposure can be helpful
- Repeat, rephrase, and summarize what has already been said
- Allow adequate time for older adults to process what was said

Discussion Questions

1. Would the use of gestures help auditory comprehension in the elderly?
2. In addition to hearing aids, what are other assistive listening devices or amplification devices that can be used by older adults?
3. How would older adults add to their vocabulary store and word-related knowledge?
4. As noted in the book, many factors affect older adults' auditory comprehension (e.g., environment, hearing loss). Is there one primary factor that contributes to these reductions in auditory comprehension?

References

American Speech-Language-Hearing Association (ASHA). (2007). *Accents and dialects.* Retrieved June 26, 2007 from http://www.asha.org/about/leadership-projects/multicultural/issues/ad

Balota, D. A., & Duchek, J. M. (1991). Semantic priming effects, lexical repetition effects, and contextual disambiguation effects in healthy aged individuals and individuals with senile dementia of the Alzheimer type. *Brain and Language, 40,* 181–201.

Bayles, K. A., & Tomoeda, C. K. (1993). *Arizona Battery for Communication Disorders of Dementia.* Tucson, AZ: Canyonlands Publishing.

Blanton, D. J., & Degenais, P. A. (2007). Comparison of language skills of adjudicated and nonadjudicated adolescent males and females. *Language, Speech, and Hearing Services in Schools, 38,* 309–314.

Burda, A. N. (2007). *Communication changes in healthy aging adults.* Adele Whitenack Davis Research in Gerontology Award, University of Northern Iowa.

Burda, A. N., Bradley-Potter, M., Dralle, J., Murphy, J., & Roehs, A. (2009). Influence of age and native language on immediate verbal repetition. *Perceptual and Motor Skills, 109,* 1–8.

Burda, A. N, Casey, A. M., Foster, T. R., Pilkington, A. K., & Reppe, E. A. (2006). Effects of accent and age on transcription of medically related utterances: A pilot study. *Communication Disorders Quarterly, 27,* 110–116.

Burda, A. N., & Hageman, C. F. (2005). Perception of accented speech by residents in assisted living facilities. *Journal of Medical Speech Language Pathology, 13,* 7–14.

Burda, A. N., Overhake, D. R., & Thompson, K. K. (2005). Familiarity and older adults' transcriptions of native and non-native speech. *Perceptual and Motor Skills, 100,* 939–942.

Burda, A. N., Scherz, J. A., Hageman, C. F., & Edwards, H. T. (2003). Effects of age on understanding speakers with Spanish or Taiwanese accents. *Perceptual and Motor Skills, 97*, 11–20.

Burke, D. M., & Harrold, R. M. (1993). Automatic and effortful semantic processes in old age: Experimental and naturalistic approaches. In L. L. Light & D. M. Burke (Eds.), *Language, memory, and aging* (pp. 100–116). New York: Cambridge University Press.

Caplan, D., & Waters, G. S. (1999). Verbal working memory and sentence comprehension. *Behavioral and Brain Sciences, 22*, 77–126.

Clarke, C. M. (2002). *Perceptual adjustment to foreign-accented English with short-term exposure.* Paper presented at the Seventh International Conference on Spoken Language Processing, Buffalo, NY.

Cohen, G., & Faulkner, D. (1986). Does "elderspeak" work? The effect of intonation and stress on comprehension and recall of spoken discourse in old age. *Language and Communication, 6*, 91–98.

Committee on Hearing, Bioacoustics, and Biomechanics. (CHABA). (1998). Speech understanding and aging. *Journal of the Acoustical Society of America, 83*, 859–895.

Corso, F. (1963). Age and sex differences in pure-tone thresholds. *Archives of Otolaryngology, 77*, 385–405.

Dubno, J. R., Ahlstrom, J. B., & Horwitz, A. R. (2000). Use of context by young and aged adults with normal hearing. *Journal of the Acoustical Society of America, 107*, 538–546.

Dugan, M. (2003). *Living with hearing loss.* Washington, DC: Gallaudet University Press.

Edwards, H. T., & Strattman, K. H. (1996). *Accent modification manual: Materials and activities; Instructor's Text.* San Diego, CA: Singular Publishing Group.

Federmeier, K. D. (2006). Thinking ahead: The role and roots of prediction in language comprehension. *Psychophysiology, 44*, 491–505.

Federmeier, K. D., & Kutas, M. (2005). Aging in context: Age-related changes in context use during language comprehension. *Psychophysiology, 42*, 133–141.

Garstecki, D. D., & Erler, S. F. (1997). Hearing in older adults. In B. B. Shadden & M. A. Toner (Eds.), *Aging and communication: For clinicians by clinicians* (pp. 97–116). Austin, TX: Pro-Ed.

Gass, S., & Varonis, E. M. (1984). The effect of familiarity on the comprehensibility of nonnative speech. *Language Learning, 34*, 65–86.

Goodglass, H., Kaplan, E., & Barresi, B. (2001). *Boston Diagnostic Aphasia Examination* (3rd ed.). Philadelphia: Lippincott Williams & Wilkins.

Gordon-Salant, S. (2005). Hearing loss and aging: New research findings and clinical implications. *Journal of Rehabilitation Research and Development, 42*, 9–24.

Gordon-Salant, S., & Fitzgibbons, P. J. (1993). Temporal factors and speech recognition performance in young and elderly listeners. *Journal of Speech and Hearing Research, 36*, 1276–1285.

Gordon-Salant, S., & Fitzgibbons, P. J. (1995). Comparing recognition of distorted speech using an equivalent signal-to-noise ratio index. *Journal of Speech and Hearing Research, 38*, 706–713.

Gordon-Salant, S., & Fitzgibbons, P. J. (1999). Profile of auditory temporal processing in older adults. *Journal of Speech, Language, and Hearing Research, 42*, 300–311.

Gordon-Salant, S., & Fitzgibbons, P. J. (2004). Effects of stimulus and noise rate variability on speech perception by younger and older adults. *Journal of the Acoustical Society of America, 115*, 1808–1117.

Helfer, K., & Wilber, L. A. (1990). Hearing loss, aging, and speech perception in rever-beration and noise. *Journal of Speech and Hearing Research, 33*, 149–155.

Helm-Estabrooks, N. (1992). *Aphasia Diagnostic Profile*. Dedham, MA: AliMed.

Humes, L. E. (1996). Speech understanding in the elderly. *Journal of the American Academy of Audiology, 7*, 161–167.

Keenan, J. S., & Brassell, E. G. (1975). *Aphasia Language Performance Scales*. Murfreesboro, TN: Pinnacle Press.

Kemper, S., & Harden, T. (1999). Experimentally disentangling what's beneficial about elderspeak from what's not. *Psychology and Aging, 14*, 656–670.

Kertesz, A. (2006). *Western Aphasia Battery–Revised*. San Antonio, TX: Harcourt Assessment, Inc.

Kjelgaard, M. M., Titone, D. A., & Wingfield, A. (1999). The influence of prosodic structure on the interpretation of temporary syntactic ambiguity by young and elderly listeners. *Experimental Aging Research, 25*, 187–207.

Light, L. L., Valencia-Laver, D., & Davis, D. (1991). Instantiation of general terms in young and older adults. *Psychology and Aging, 6*, 337–351.

Little, D. M., Prentice, K. J., Darrow, A. W., & Wingfield, A. (2005). Listening to spo-ken text: Adult age differences as revealed by self-paced listening. *Experimental Aging Research, 31*, 313–330.

Lipsky, M., & King, M. (2005). *Blueprints family medicine* (2nd ed.). Malden, MA: Lippincott Williams & Wilkins.

Major, R. C., Fitzmaurice, S. F., Bunta, F., & Balasubramanian, C. (2002). The effects of non-native accents on listening comprehension: Implications for ESL assessment. *TESOL Quarterly, 2*, 173–190.

Markowitz, J. (2008). Evidence-based psychotherapies for depression. *Journal of Occupational and Environmental Medicine, 50*, 437–440.

Martin, F. N., & Greer Clark, J. (2006). *Introduction to audiology* (9th ed.). Boston: Pearson.

Mehrotra, C., & Wagner, L. (2008). *Aging and diversity: An active learning experience* (2nd ed.). New York: CRC Press.

Meyers, P. S. (1999). *Right hemisphere damage: Disorders of communication and cognition*. San Diego, CA: Singular Publishing Group.

Munro, M. J., & Derwing, T. M. (1995a). Foreign accent, comprehensibility and intel-ligibility in the speech of second language learners. *Language Learning, 45*, 73–97.

Munro, M. J., & Derwing, T. M. (1995b). Processing time, accent, and comprehensi-bility in the perception of native and foreign-accented speech. *Language and Speech, 38*, 289–306.

Nabelek, A. K., & Robinson, P. K. (1982). Monaural and binaural speech perception in reverberation for listeners of various ages. *Journal of the Acoustical Society of America, 71*, 1242–1248.

Nejime, Y., & Moore, B. C. (1998). Evaluation of the effect of speech-rate slowing on speech intelligibility in noise using a simulation of cochlear hearing loss. *Journal of the Acoustical Society of America, 103*, 572–576.

Pichora-Fuller, M. K. (2008). Use of supportive context by younger and older adult listeners: Balancing bottom-up and top-down information processing. *International Journal of Audiology, 47*, S72–S82.

Pichora-Fuller, M. K., Schneider, B. A., & Daneman, M. (1995). How young and old adults listen to and remember speech in noise. *Journal of the Acoustical Society of America, 97*, 593–608.

Powell, J. A., Hale, M. A., & Bayer, A. J. (1995). Symptoms of communication break-down in dementia: Carers' perceptions. *European Journal of Disorders of Communication,* 30, 65–75.

Salthouse, T. A. (1993). Effects of aging on verbal abilities: Examination of the psy-chometric literature. In L. L. Lights & D. M. Burke (Eds.), *Language, memory, and aging* (pp. 17–35). New York: Cambridge University Press.

Santo Pietro, M . J., & Ostuni, E. (2003). *Successful communication with Alzheimer's disease patients: An in-service manual* (2nd ed.). Newton, MA: Butterworth–Heinemann.

Schmitt, J. F., & Moore, J. R. (1989). Natural alteration of speaking rate: The effect of passage comprehension by listeners over 75 years of age. *Journal of Speech and Hearing Research,* 32, 445–450.

Schneider, B. A., Daneman, M., & Murphy, D. R. (2005). Speech comprehension dif-ficulties in older adults: Cognitive slowing or age-related changes in hearing? *Psychology and Aging,* 20, 261–271.

Schneider, B. A., Daneman, M., Murphy, D. R., & Kwong-See, S. (2000). Listening to discourse in distracting settings: The effects of aging. *Psychology and Aging,* 15, 110–125.

Schneider, B., Daneman, M., & Pichora-Fuller, M. K. (2002). Listening in aging adults: From discourse comprehension to psychoacoustics. *Canadian Journal of Experimental Psychology,* 56, 139–152.

Soederberg Miller, L. M., Stine-Morrow, E. A. L., Kirkorian, H. L., & Conroy, M. L. (2004). Age differences in knowledge-driven reading. *Journal of Educational Psychology,* 96, 811–821.

Thornton, R., & Light, L. L. (2006). Language comprehension and production in normal aging. In J. E. Birren & K. W. Schaie (Eds.), *Handbook of the psychology of aging* (6th ed., pp. 261–287). San Diego, CA: Elsevier.

Tun, P. A. (1998). Fast noisy speech: Age differences in processing rapid speech with background noise. *Psychology and Aging,* 13, 424–434.

Tye-Murray, N. (2004). *Foundations of aural rehabilitation: Children, adults, and their family mem-bers* (2nd ed.). Clifton Park, NY: Delmar Learning.

van Rooij, J. C. G. M., & Plomp, M. (1990). Auditive and cognitive factors in speech perception in elderly listeners. II: Multivariate analyses. *Journal of the Acoustical Society of America,* 88, 2611–2624.

Wennerstrom, A. (2001). *The music of everyday speech: Prosody and discourse analysis.* New York: Oxford Press.

Willott, J. F. (1991). *Aging and the auditory system: Anatomy, physiology, and psychophysics.* San Diego, CA: Singular.

Wingfield, A., Alexander, A. H., & Cavigelli, S. (1994). Does memory constrain utiliza-tion of top-down information in spoken word recognition? Evidence from nor-mal aging. *Language and Speech,* 37, 221–235.

Wingfield, A., Lahar, C. J., & Stine, E. A. L. (1989). Age and decision strategies in run-ning memory for speech: Effects of prosody and linguistic structure. *Journal of Gerontology: Psychological Sciences,* 44, P106–P113.

Wingfield, A., Lindfield, K., & Goodglass, H. (2000). Effects of age and hearing sen-sitivity on the use of prosodic information in spoken word recognition. *Journal of Speech, Language, and Hearing Research,* 43, 915–925.

Wingfield, A., Poon, L. W., Lombardi, L., & Lowe, D. (1985). Speed of processing in normal aging: Effects of speech rate, linguistic structure, and processing time. *Journal of Gerontology,* 40, 579–585.

Wingfield, A., Wayland, S. C., & Stine, E. A. L. (1992). Adult age differences in the use of prosody for syntactic parsing and recall of spoken sentences. *Journal of Gerontology: Psychological Sciences, 47,* P350–P356.

Yonan, C. A., & Sommers, M. S. (2000). The effects of talker familiarity on spoken word identification in younger and older listeners. *Psychology and Aging, 14,* 88–99.

Yorkston, K. M., & Beukelman, D. R. (1984). *Assessment of intelligibility of dysarthric speech.* Austin, TX: Pro-Ed.

Yost, W. (2007). *Fundamentals of hearing: An introduction* (5th ed.). Burlington, MA: Academic Press.

Chapter 4

Reading Comprehension

Angela N. Burda, PhD, CCC-SLP

Jill L. Champley, PhD, CCC-SLP

Introduction

Reading allows us to gain knowledge and, for many, engage in an enjoyable leisure activity (McEvoy & Vincent, 1980). Older adults, in particular, report that they enjoy reading (Boulton-Lewis, Buys, & Kitchin, 2006; Peppers, 1976). The breadth of reading skills is wide ranging, requiring systematic application of meaning to strings of letters (Beeson & Hillis, 2008). For example, we can read and understand information from a large range of sources, such as books and magazines, food and beverage selections found on menus, and the instructions for medications. For aging adults, adequate reading comprehension abilities are increasingly necessary as they learn to use new technology and have greater access to healthcare information and complex personal finance management systems (De Beni, Palladino, Borella, & Lo Presti, 2002; Harris, Rogers, & Qualls, 1998). Reading requires the rapid recognition of semantic and orthographic input (Carlisle, 2003; Kamhi & Catts, 1999; Nagy, Anderson, Schommer, Scott, & Stallman, 1989; Napps, 1989). Aspects of cognition can also factor into reading comprehension

(Daneman & Carpenter, 1980; Qualls & Harris, 2003; see Chapter 2 on cognition). This is not surprising, because if individuals cannot retain what they have read, their understanding will be reduced. There are also various theoretical perspectives to keep in mind regarding age-related changes in comprehension abilities (see Chapter 1 on theoretical perspectives). People do not typically contemplate the reading process until difficulties occur.

This chapter will discuss what aging adults' reading comprehension abilities generally should be, factors that can negatively affect older adults' reading comprehension, signs that may warrant referral to a speech-language pathologist or other medical professionals, and what strategies can help maintain or improve aging adults' reading comprehension. A list of "Quick Facts" at the end of the chapter summarizes important points.

Older Adults' General Reading Comprehension Abilities

Speech-language pathologists (SLPs) who work with adults must evaluate their patients' language comprehension and expression. Assessment tools divide these broad language areas into subtests (e.g., Reading Comprehension, Writing) and, in many cases, arrange items in a hierarchical manner. Thus, subtests begin with directions and/or responses that are shorter and simpler in nature and progress to lengthier, more complex items (LaPointe & Horner, 1998). In several of the commercially available tests for adults, reading-comprehension tasks generally involve: matching words and sentences to pictures, choosing the correct word to complete a sentence, selecting the appropriate information to complete a questionnaire, following written commands, answering questions after reading sentences and stories, and answering questions pertaining to functional reading materials (e.g., labels on pill bottles) (Bayles & Tomoeda, 1993; Helm-Estabrooks, 1992; Kertesz, 2006; LaPointe & Horner, 1998; Schuell, 1973).

Finding information about neurologically intact aging adults' reading comprehension abilities can be challenging. Research studies have not necessarily included clinical tasks found in speech-language pathology tests, such as those previously mentioned (e.g., matching words to pictures). Not all tests have systematically included aging adults as part of the standardization process or reported the ages of the normal adults in the assessment manuals (Schuell, 1973). In certain cases, the normal group could be considered questionable. For example, as discussed in Chapter 3, the normal group in the standardization study for the *Aphasia Language Performance Scale* (ALPS) was composed solely of prisoners (Keenan & Brassell, 1975). The authors reported that they wanted to find participants that roughly estimated the abilities of Veterans Administration patients, which in their opinion, included persons who were neither highly educated nor intelligent. Although including adults who represent a variety of socioeconomic status and intellectual levels would be helpful as part of test standardization, including incarcerated individuals would not give a good example of normal language performance because many in the penal system have documented language disorders (Blanton & Degenais, 2007). When tests have included normal aging adults, these older individuals have not necessarily been a separate control group. Some exceptions exist, and information found in test manuals, coupled with empirical data in the literature, can provide a general guide of what the normal reading comprehension abilities are for neurologically intact older adults.

As described in Chapter 3, two tests, the *Aphasia Diagnostic Profile* (ADP; Helm-Estabrooks, 1992) and the *Arizona Battery for Communication Disorders of Dementia* (ABCD; Bayles & Tomoeda, 1993), included older adults as part of the standardization process. The ADP included data from 40 neurologically intact adults aged 20–99 years. Although 11 of these adults fell within the age range of 60–99, the test's author did not report the normative data by specific age groups. The ADP's Reading subtest requires individuals to read and respond to a patient information sheet. The first section of this subtest asks for biographical information in a fill-in-the-blank format (e.g., name, address). The second section includes questions such as their age range, marital status, and number of children. Patients then select the appropriate response. The ADP's test manual reports that neurologically intact adults in their standardization study had a mean score of 22.4 ($SD = 13.1$) out of a total of 30 points possible, or 75% correct. A multidimensional scoring system is used for many subtests of the ADP, and the immediacy of a response is included as part of this scoring system. Although not reported in the test manual, it is possible that the normal adults were able to understand what they read and select the correct answer but were slow to respond, which would result in a lower score.

The ABCD (Bayles & Tomoeda, 1993) is one of the few tests in which older adults in the standardization research were a separate control group. Its Reading Comprehension subtest was designed to assess understanding at both word and sentence levels. For the word level, persons must select one picture out of the four presented that matches a written word (e.g., bugs, policeman, waiting). For the sentence level, individuals read a sentence (e.g., "The boy is throwing the ball") and then select the correct answer to a single question (e.g., "What did he throw?"). Four possible answers are presented (e.g., a bell, some balls, a ball, the boy). On the word-picture matching task, older adults in the standardization sample ($M_{age} = 70.44$ years, $SD = 17.07$) scored a mean of 7.9 correct ($SD = 0.7$) out of a total of 8 items possible, or 99% correct. This score did not differ significantly from that of a group of normal young adults who were also included as part of the standardization sample. For the sentences, the neurologically intact aging adults had a mean score of 6.4 ($SD = 0.5$) correct out of a total of 7 items possible, or 91% correct. This score was slightly lower than that of the normal young adults, who had a mean score of 6.9 ($SD = 0.3$) on this subtest, or 99% correct.

In addition to information from standardized tests, investigations have been conducted on older adults' reading abilities. Word-level comprehension does not appear to change with age (Stine-Morrow, Milinder, Pullara, & Herman, 2001); however, findings on sentence comprehension are ambiguous. Some researchers have found that older adults have good comprehension and recall of sentences, others have reported that older adults have difficulties with such tasks (Stine-Morrow, Milinder, et al., 2001). Studies on reading speed indicate that older adults typically read printed materials and online information at a slower pace compared with younger adults (Connelly, Hasher, & Zacks, 1991; Hartley, Stojack, Mushaney, Kiku Annon, & Lee, 1994).

More recently, reading-related abilities have been investigated in the aging population. A study by Champley (2005) measured decoding, vocabulary, phonological awareness, and morphological awareness abilities in adults aged 65 and older. Decoding was measured by having participants complete the Word Attack and Word Identification subtests of the *Woodcock Reading Mastery Tests–Revised* (Woodcock, 1998). For the Word Identification subtest, individuals produced a "natural reading" of a given word regardless of their knowledge of the word's meaning. The Word Attack subtest required participants to read nonsense words or words with a low frequency of occurrence. For both subtests, the normed mean was 100 ($SD = 15$). Older adults achieved a mean standard score of 106.78 ($SD = 10.26$) on the Word Identification subtest and a mean standard score of 102.27 ($SD = 11.02$) on the Word Attack subtest. Both scores were slightly above the reported mean. Champley (2005) then measured reading vocabulary using the vocabulary subtest of the *Nelson-Denny Reading Test* (Brown, Fishco, & Hanna, 1993). Participants had 15 minutes to respond to multiple-choice items describing the meaning of given words. Normalized scale scores were used, and out of a total 258 possible, older adults had a mean normalized scale score of 241.98 ($SD = 18.96$).

Phonological awareness encompasses the abilities to manipulate both individual sounds and words using various activities, such as rhyming or segmenting words into individual sounds (National Institute for Literacy, 2003). To assess phonological awareness, Champley (2005) administered two nonstandardized measures designed by Moran and Fitch (2001). In the Phoneme-Switching task, aging adults listened to two words in which the initial sound of each word was reversed and then were asked to state the target phrase within seven seconds (e.g., for "dasta pish," the participant would say "pasta dish"). The Phonetic-Reversal task consisted of words that when pronounced backwards made a different word. Older adults listened to the item and then stated the correct word within three seconds (e.g., "kiss" backwards is "sick"). Raw scores were reported with a total of 20 points possible for each subtest. On the Phoneme-Switching task, older adults obtained a mean score of 9.15 (SD = 6.54), or 46% accuracy. For the Phonetic-Reversal task, aging adults had a mean score of 6.42 (SD = 5.68), or 32% correct. In general, the participants had considerable variability in their performance on these two tasks. The time constraints associated with both tasks may have contributed to the older adults' overall low mean performance.

Champley (2005) used two measures to assess older adults' morphological awareness, which is the ability to use the knowledge of word meanings to spell and comprehend words. The first was a modified version of the *Test of Morphological Structure* (TMS; Carlisle, 2000). Participants were presented with a target base word (e.g., *rely, major*) followed by an incomplete sentence. They then generated a derived form of the base word (e.g., *reliably, majority*) to complete the sentence within three seconds. The second morphological task, the "Comes From" task (Katz, 2004; Nagy, Berninger, Abbott, Vaughan, & Vermeulen, 2003), is a non-standardized measure that has a list of word pairs in which there could be orthographic and/or phonological changes between the base word and the target word. Participants decided whether or not the first word in the pair came from the second word (e.g., *teacher-teach, single-sing*). Raw scores were obtained for both of these tasks, and similar to the phonological awareness measures, each had a total of 20 points possible. For the TMS, the older adults achieved a mean score of 18.28 (SD = 2.82), or 91% accuracy. For the "Comes From" task, participants obtained a mean score of 19.06 (SD = 1.12), or 95% accuracy.

In the 2007 study conducted by Burda described in Chapter 3 (in which 31 adults aged 65 and older were divided into three age categories: Young-Old, Middle-Old, and Old-Old), participants were required to complete a variety of reading-comprehension tasks that could be clinically evaluated by SLPs. These tasks included having participants match words to pictures, match sentences to pictures, select the word that best completed a sentence, and answer wh-questions after hearing a short story (seven sentences long) about a man vacuuming. Participants were also asked to answer wh-questions after reading a grocery store advertisement (e.g., "How much does a pound of hamburger cost?"), a gas bill (e.g., "When is the payment due?"), and a phone message that a son took for his mother (e.g., "Who is the message for?"). Results of this study are included in **Table 4-1**, broken down by age groups.

Table 4-1

Mean Performance for Reading-Comprehension Tasks

Task	Total*	Young-Old			Middle-Old			Old-Old		
		M	SD	%**	M	SD	%**	M	SD	%**
Match words to pictures	10	10.0	0.0	100	10.0	0.0	100	10.0	0.0	100
Match sentence to pictures	10	10.0	0.0	100	9.8	0.6	98	9.9	0.3	99
Sentence completion	10	8.2	1.2	82	8.7	1.5	87	8.9	1.4	89
Short story wh- Qs	10	9.7	0.5	97	9.5	0.8	95	9.6	0.7	96
Grocery store ad	10	9.7	0.7	97	8.8	1.5	88	9.8	0.4	98
Gas bill	10	8.4	1.1	84	7.6	1.5	76	7.2	1.8	72
Message for mom	10	8.8	1.1	88	8.6	1.0	86	8.6	1.2	86

Note: *refers to the total number of points possible. **refers to the percentage correct.
Source: Burda (2007).

As shown in Table 4-1, participants had high accuracy levels for most tasks. Older adults garnered the highest scores for matching words and sentences to pictures, answering questions after reading a short story, and answering questions pertaining to a grocery advertisement. They had lower scores on the sentence-completion task, answering questions from the "Message for Mom," and in particular, when answering questions related to a gas bill. Poorer performance on the gas bill may have been related to the overall readability of the document. Information was not as easy to find, and the print size was smaller on the gas bill compared with the grocery store ad. With the exception of the gas bill, no marked differences occurred across age groups. In fact, on the sentence-completion and grocery-ad tasks, the Old-Old group had higher mean scores than participants in the two younger age groups. In addition, no statistically significant differences occurred in performance among the three age groups. It should be noted that the sample size for this pilot study was small.

In summary, based on information included in the normative data for adult language tests and in research studies, older adults should be able to accurately match words and sentences to pictures, and answer wh-questions after reading a single sentence or short story. While they should be able to select answers to a personal information questionnaire, choose a word to complete a written sentence, and answer questions related to functional reading materials, their performance scores on these tasks may be lower or more variable compared with the previously mentioned tasks. Older adults read more slowly than younger adults, both when reading printed text and online materials. They demonstrate poor performance and significant variability on phonological-awareness tasks; however, time constraints associated with such tests may negatively impact their scores. Older adults do well on meas-ures of decoding, reading vocabulary, and morphological awareness. It is important to bear in mind that neurologically intact adults may be able to do far more than is reported here, as this information is based on only a limited amount of available data. More research is needed to better document these abilities.

Factors Affecting Older Adults' Reading Comprehension and Signs of Problems

Several factors can adversely affect older adults' reading comprehension. The presence of any of these factors can also lead to poorer performance on tests frequently used with older adults, such as the Mini-Mental State Examination (Folstein, Folstein, & Fanjiang, 2001; Mayeaux et al., 1995). Many of these issues overlap with one another. For example, adults aged 75 and older read less than those aged 65–74. This change in reading habits may be related to declines in health, increases in sensory distur-bances, and/or cohort differences in educational levels (Fisher, 1986). Vision is one area that undergoes significant change. As the lens of the eye becomes more opaque and begins to yellow with age, less light reaches the retina (Smith, 1993). As a result, older adults have greater difficulty with visual acuity and accommodation. Visual acuity is the eye's abil-ity to differentiate fine details such as small print, while visual accom-modation refers to the ability of the lens to adjust its shape in order to bring distant objects into focus (Smith, 1993). Aging adults exhibit re-duced contrast sensitivity (Rubin, Roche, Prasada-Rao, & Fried, 1994) and develop presbyopia, the age-related decline in the ability to see close up. Older adults' visual field is also reduced, making it difficult for them to see adequately in low levels of light (Fozard, Wolf, Bell, McFarland, & Podolsky, 1977). Such visual changes can make reading more challenging.

The effects of cognitive functioning and verbal skills on older adults' reading abilities have been studied. Individuals who have larger working memory capacities and/or higher levels of vocabulary can re-call more of the information they have read (Stine-Morrow, Loveless, & Soederberg, 1996; Stine-Morrow, Miller, & Leno, 2001). Aging adults who are considered good readers have higher verbal abilities (Meyer, Young, & Bartlett, 1989), and possessing these skills coupled with reading strate-gies may offset age-related reading difficulties (Stine-Morrow, Milinder et al., 2001). Many researchers, however, report that working memory reductions in older adults lead to poorer reading abilities (De Beni et al., 2002; Meyer, Marsiske, & Willis, 1993; Smiler, Gagne, & Stine-Morrow, 2003; Waters & Caplan, 2001), such as greater difficultly comprehending syntactically complex forms (Kemper, 1987). Adults over the age of 85 have been found to have the greatest declines with working memory

(De Beni et al., 2002). The ability to rapidly process written information appears to slow with age (Gausman Benson & Forman, 2002), and aging adults are generally more distractible than younger adults (Meyer, Marsiske, & Willis, 1993). Thus, older adults take more time and use more effort when reading (Smiler et al., 2003).

Health, educational level, and employment can also factor into older adults' reading abilities. Those in poorer health have greater difficulty reading (Dewalt, Berkman, Sheridan, Lohr, & Pignone, 2004; Weiss, Hart, McGee, & D'Estelle, 1992) and are less likely to read than their healthy peers (Fisher, 1986). Older adults with higher levels of education tend to have better reading comprehension abilities (Gausman Benson & Forman, 2002), while those identified as having poor reading comprehension or as nonreaders (i.e., they have not read any books, newspapers, or magazines within the past six months) typically have less education (De Beni et al., 2002: Gazmararian et al., 1999; McEvoy & Vincent, 1980). The current cohort of older adults may have less formal education than subsequent generations (McEvoy & Vincent, 1980) because many left school at a young age to join the military (Elder, 1986). Reading abilities also tend to be higher in aging adults who are either employed or actively volunteer (National Center for Education Statistics, 1999).

The type of reading materials and the organization of the passage can affect older adults' comprehension. Aging adults have difficulty understanding health-related information, including instructions for a medical procedure, a Medicaid application, directions on a pill bottle, and informed consent forms (Gausman Benson & Forman, 2002). Such struggles can have dire consequences such as older adults' failure to take their medications as prescribed. Some studies indicate that aging adults have better understanding of expository passages (e.g., newspapers) compared with narrative passages (Champley, Scherz, Apel, & Burda, 2008; Harris et al., 1998; Zelinski & Gilewski, 1988). These findings may be in part due to their prior knowledge (Leslie & Caldwell, 2001) as well as their regular exposure to expository texts (Smith, 1993, 1996). A recent study exploring older adults' reading comprehension used an expository passage that described ultrasound and a narrative passage about Andrew Carnegie (Champley et al., 2008). Participants scored higher on the expository passage, possibly because some of them may have had previous experience with ultrasound. Older adults also tend to frequently read newspapers and magazines, making them familiar with this genre (Champley et al., 2008; Smith, 1993, 1996). Not all researchers have found similar results. One study reported that adults aged 70 and older had adequate reading comprehension of narrative passages but had significant difficulty understanding expository text (De Beni et al., 2002). If reading passages are not well organized in a manner that older adults can easily identify or utilize, they will likely have poorer comprehension and recall (Meyer, 1987; Yussen &

Glysch, 1993). Certain types of reading materials generally adhere to specific types of organizational structures. For example, historical passages tend to follow a time-ordered sequence, while scientific articles present background information on a problem and then provide potential solutions (Meyer, 1987).

Despite age-related declines in cognitive and perceptual abilities, the majority of older adults should not have extensive struggles with reading and should be able to continue with everyday reading tasks (De Beni et al., 2002; Smith, 1993). There are signs, however, that can indicate they are having reading difficulties and should be referred to a speech-language pathologist or other medical professionals. Obviously, overt complaints of not remembering what they have read or of not being able to see or read would warrant a referral to a physician and possibly a speech-language pathologist and an optometrist. Even if aging adults do not complain about such difficulties, they can still evidence problems with reading. For example, if they are having increasing difficulty answering questions pertaining to recently read information (e.g., newspaper or magazine articles, books), they would benefit from being seen by the previously mentioned healthcare professionals. Acquired errors in oral reading or when sounding out words can be a sign of potential neurological damage (Hillis & Tuffiash, 2002). Any alteration in reading habits can also indicate problems. If older adults quit reading, it can be a sign of vision problems or may indicate that they are depressed and no longer have interest in previously enjoyed activities (Smith, 1993).

Strategies to Help Older Adults' Reading Comprehension

Several strategies can enhance aging adults' reading comprehension. First and foremost, vision problems need to be addressed. In addition, the reading environment should be as optimal as possible. Specifically, distractions should be minimized (Connelly et al., 1991) and reading areas should have proper lighting (Smith, 1993). While it is obvious that too little light will not be helpful, too much light can lead to problems with glare (Smith, 1993). Using magnifying glasses and having larger-print reading materials can be beneficial (Becker, Hans-Werner, Schilling, & Burmedi, 2005). Older adults should also be allowed as much time as possible to read so they can adequately comprehend the target information (De Beni et al., 2002; Meyer, 1987).

Teaching older adults to use specific strategies can improve their reading comprehension. Potentially effective strategies include: associating what they are reading with prior knowledge they have, deciding ahead of time on what the purpose is for reading the specific material, making predictions about what is being read, checking for a consistency of ideas throughout the passage, and using words around the text to help determine what an unknown word is (Miholic, 1994). Learning to identify and use the organization of the text can also aid comprehension and recall (Meyer, 1987). To use previously presented examples, if older adults are reading historical passages, they can learn that such information should be presented in a chronological manner. When reading scientific articles, they should expect that background information on a problem is presented first and that solutions for the problem will follow (Meyer, 1987). For newspaper articles, aging adults should anticipate that the articles will provide the details of who, where, when, and how (Meyer, 1987). Older adults tend to reread an entire passage over in order to clarify information (Champley et al., 2008). While this strategy can be beneficial, it may at times be inefficient (Zabrucky & Moore, 1994). Thus, they can also be educated to selectively reread those sections they are having difficulty understanding or remembering (Zabrucky & Moore, 1994). Using memory strategies may also help (Smith, 1993). For example, older adults can write down main ideas and/or details of what they are reading or mentally rehearse the information they wish to recall.

Another way that aging adults can aid their reading comprehension is simply by continuing to read. Continual involvement in reading may help them remain mentally active and alert and delay any possible age-related declines (Harvey & Dutton, 1979; Smith, 1993). This can be accomplished by having older adults engage in a variety of reading activities. Some may choose to read expository materials such as newspapers and news-type magazines that contain informative and relatively brief articles that can be read quickly (Champley, 2005). Others may prefer to read novels or religious materials (Herzog, Kahn, Morgan, Jackson, & Antonucci, 1989). Utilizing computers can also be beneficial since aging adults who read online reportedly are better at recalling information that they have read and identifying any inconsistencies in the text (Moore & Zabrucky, 1995). Another possibility is for older adults to continue their education. Taking classes or participating in activities such as Elderhostel or other similar lifelong learning institutes (Burda & Kuker, 2008; Jamieson, 2007) will expose them to a wide variety of reading materials and activities (Smith, 1993).

Quick Facts

- General Reading Abilities of Neurologically Intact Older Adults:
  - Accurately match words and sentences to pictures
  - Accurately answer wh- questions after reading a single sentence or a short story

- May demonstrate lower performance or more variable performance when asked to:
  - Select answers to complete a personal information questionnaire
  - Choose a word to complete a sentence
  - Answer questions related to functional reading materials
- Read printed and online materials more slowly compared with young adults
- Display poor performance and significant variability on phonological-awareness tasks possibly because of time constraints associated with such tasks
- Do well on measures of decoding, reading vocabulary, and morphological awareness
- In general, should be able to continue with everyday reading tasks
- Factors That Can Negatively Affect Older Adults' Reading:
  - Changes in vision, including:
    - Difficulty with visual acuity and visual accommodation
    - Development of presbyopia
    - Struggle with seeing in low levels of light
  - Reduced working memory capacities
  - Slowed ability to process written information
  - Distracted more easily
  - Lower verbal abilities
  - Poor health
  - Lower levels of education
  - Unemployed and/or not actively participating in volunteer work
  - Types of reading materials:
    - Health-related information is difficult for many aging adults
    - Expository reading passages (e.g., newspapers, magazines) may be easier to understand than narrative passages
  - Reading passages that are not well organized
- Signs That an Older Adult Should Be Referred to a Speech-Language Pathologist or Other Medical Professionals:
  - Overt complaints of not being able to remember what they have read or being unable to see or read
  - Frequent difficulty with answering questions pertaining to reading materials
  - Acquired errors in oral reading or when sounding out words
  - Any alteration in reading habits, such as no longer reading or reading significantly less than usual

(*Note*: If compromised vision is suspected, refer individual to an optometrist.)

- Strategies That Can Help Older Adults' Reading Abilities:
  - Address vision problems
  - Minimize distractions in the reading environment
  - Ensure adequate lighting; however, too much light can lead to glare
  - Provide a magnifying glass
  - Provide larger-print reading materials
  - Allow older adults as much time as needed to read
  - Train older adults to use these techniques to improve reading comprehension:
    - Associate what they are reading with information they already know
    - Decide ahead of time on what the purpose is for reading the specific material
    - Make predictions about what is being read
    - Check for consistency of ideas throughout the passage
    - Use words around the text to help determine an unknown word
    - Learn to identify the organization of the text:
      - Historical passages should be presented in a chronological manner
      - Scientific articles should first present background information on a problem and then provide solutions for the problem
      - Newspaper articles should provide the details of who, where, when, and how
    - Selectively reread sections that are difficult to comprehend or recall, or reread the entire passage
    - Use memory strategies, such as writing down or mentally rehearsing main ideas and/or details of the reading passage
    - Read materials online
    - Continue to engage in reading
  - Encourage older adults to seek out educational opportunities, such as taking classes or being involved in Elderhostel or other similar lifelong learning institutes

Discussion Questions

1. What aspects of cognition can affect older adults' reading comprehension?
2. Why would using the computer help aging adults with their reading?

3. What kind of information is available discussing the success of older adults who become literate later in life?
4. Because difficulty understanding health-related information can have dire consequences, what can be done to address these challenges?

References

Bayles, K. A., & Tomoeda, C. K. (1993). *Arizona Battery for Communication Disorders of Dementia.* Tucson, AZ: Canyonlands Publishing.

Becker, S., Hans-Werner, W., Schilling, O., & Burmedi, D. (2005). Assistive device use in visually impaired older adults: Role of control beliefs. *Gerontologist, 45, 739–746.*

Beeson, P. M., & Hillis, A. E. (2008). Comprehension and production of written words. In R. Chapey (Ed.), *Language intervention strategies in aphasia and related neurogenic communication disorders* (5th ed., pp. 654–688). Baltimore, MD: Lippincott, Williams, & Wilkins.

Blanton, D. J., & Degenais, P. A. (2007). Comparison of language skills of adjudicated and nonadjudicated adolescent males and females. *Language, Speech, and Hearing Services in Schools, 38, 309–314.*

Boulton-Lewis, G. M., Buys, L., & Kitchin, J. L. (2006). Learning and active aging. *Educational Gerontology, 32, 271–282.*

Burda, A. N. (2007). *Communication changes in healthy aging adults.* Adele Whitenack Davis Research in Gerontology Award, University of Northern Iowa.

Burda, A. N., & Kuker, L. M. (2008). Communication changes in aging adults: Impact for lifelong learning. *Conference Proceedings of the Hawaii International Education Conference, 6,* 4656–4662.

Brown, J. I., Fishco, V. V., & Hanna, G. (1993). *Nelson-Denny Reading Test.* Itasca, IL: Riverside.

Carlisle, J. F. (2000). Awareness of the structure and meaning of morphologically complex words: Impact on reading. *Reading and Writing: An Interdisciplinary Journal, 12,* 169–190.

Carlisle, J. F. (2003). Morphology matters in learning to read: A commentary. *Reading Psychology, 24, 291–322.*

Champley, J. L. (2005). *An analysis of reading materials and strategies used by older adults.* Unpublished doctoral dissertation, Wichita State University, Kansas.

Champley, J., Scherz, J. W., Apel, K., & Burda, A. (2008). A preliminary analysis of reading materials and strategies used by older adults. *Communication Disorders Quarterly, 29,* 131–140.

Connelly, L. S., Hasher, L., & Zacks, R. T. (1991). Age and reading: The impact of distraction. *Psychology and Aging, 6,* 533–541.

Daneman, M., & Carpenter, P. A. (1980). Individual differences in working memory and reading. *Journal of Verbal Learning and Verbal Behavior, 19,* 450–460.

De Beni, R., Palladino, P., Borella, E., & Lo Presti, S. (2002). Reading comprehension and aging: Does an age-related difference necessarily mean impairment? *Aging Clinical and Experimental Research, 15,* 67–76.

Dewalt, D. A., Berkman, N. D., Sheridan, S., Lohr, K. N., & Pignone, M. P. (2004). Literacy and health outcomes: A systematic review of literature. *Journal of General Internal Medicine, 19,* 228–239.

Elder, G. H. (1986). Military times and turning points in men's lives. *Developmental Psychology, 22,* 233–245.

Fisher, J. (1986). Literacy usage among older adults. In K. Landers (Ed.), *Proceedings for the Annual Adult Educational Research Conference* (pp. 94–99). Syracuse, NY: ERIC Document Reproduction Service, No. ED 269 571.

Folstein, M. F., Folstein, S. E., & Fanjiang, G. (2001). *Mini-mental state examination: Clinical guide.* Lutz, FL: Psychological Assessment Resources, Inc.

Fozard, J. L., Wolf, E., Bell, B., McFarland, R. A., & Podolsky, S. (1977). Visual perception and communication. In J. E. Birren & K. W. Schaie (Eds.), *Handbook of the psychology of aging* (pp. 497–534). New York: Van Nostrand Reinhold.

Gausman Benson, J., & Forman, W. B. (2002). Comprehension of written health care information in an affluent geriatric retirement community: Use of the Test of Functional Health Literacy. *Gerontology, 48,* 93–97.

Gazmararian, J. A., Baker, D. W., Williams, M. V., Parker, R. M., Green, D., Scott, T. et al. (1999). Health literacy among Medicare enrollees in a managed care organization. *Journal of the American Medical Association, 281,* 545–551.

Harris, J. L., Rogers, W. A., & Qualls, C. D. (1998). Written language comprehension in younger and older adults. *Journal of Speech, Language, and Hearing Research, 41,* 603–617.

Hartley, J. T., Stojack, C. C., Mushaney, T. J., Kiku Annon, T. A., & Lee, D. W. (1994). Reading speed and prose memory in older and younger adults. *Psychology and Aging, 9,* 216–223.

Harvey, R. L., & Dutton, D. (1979). Reading interests of older adults. *Educational Gerontology, 4,* 209–214.

Helm-Estabrooks, N. (1992). *Aphasia Diagnostic Profile.* Dedham, MA: AliMed.

Herzog, A., Kahn, R., Morgan, J., Jackson, J., & Antonucci, T. (1989). Age differences in productive activities. *Journal of Gerontology, 44,* S129–S138.

Hillis, A. E., & Tuffiash, E. (2002). Neuroanatomical aspects of reading. In A. Hillis (Ed.), *The handbook of adult language disorders: Integrating cognitive neuropsychology, neurology, and rehabilitation* (pp. 15–25). New York: Psychology Press.

Jamieson, A. (2007). Higher education in later life: What is the point? *Aging and Society, 27,* 363–384.

Kamhi, A. G., & Catts. H. W. (1999). Language and reading: Convergences and divergences. In H. W. Catts & A. G. Kamhi (Eds.), *Language and reading disabilities* (pp. 1–24). Boston, MA: Allyn & Bacon.

Katz, L. A. (2004). *An investigation of morphological awareness to reading comprehension in fourth and sixth graders.* Unpublished doctoral dissertation, University of Michigan, Ann Arbor, MI.

Keenan, J. S., & Brassell, E. G. (1975). *Aphasia Language Performance Scales.* Murfreesboro, TN: Pinnacle Press.

Kemper, S. (1987). Syntactic complexity and elderly adults' prose recall. *Experimental Aging Research, 13,* 47–52.

Kertesz, A. (2006). *Western Aphasia Battery–Revised.* San Antonio, TX: Harcourt Assessment, Inc.

LaPointe, J. L., & Horner, J. (1998). *Reading Comprehension Battery for Aphasia* (2nd ed.). Austin, TX: Pro-Ed.

Leslie, L., & Caldwell, J. (2001). *Qualitative Reading Inventory–3.* New York: Longman.

Mayeaux, E. J. Jr., Davis, T. C., Jackson, R. H., Henry, D., Patton, P., Slay, L., & Sentell, T. (1995). Literacy and self-reported educational levels in relation to Mini-Mental State Examination scores. *Family Medicine Journal, 27,* 658–662.

McEvoy, G., & Vincent, C. (1980). Who reads and why. *Journal of Communication, 30,* 134–140.

Meyer, B. J. F. (1987). Reading comprehension and aging. *Annual Review of Gerontology and Geriatrics, 7,* 93–115.

Meyer, B. J. F., Marsiske, M., & Willis, S. L. (1993). Text processing variables predict the readability of everyday documents read by older adults. *Reading Research Quarterly, 28*, 234–249.

Meyer, B. J. F., Young, C. J., & Bartlett, B. J. (1989). *Memory improved: Reading and memory enhancement across the life span through strategic text structures.* Hillsdale, NJ: Lawrence Erlbaum Associates.

Miholic, V. (1994). An inventory to pique students' metacognitive awareness of reading strategies. *Journal of Reading, 38*, 84–86.

Moore, D., & Zabrucky, K. (1995). Adult age differences in comprehension and memory for computer-displayed and printed text. *Educational Gerontology, 21*, 139–150.

Moran, M. J., & Fitch, J. L. (2001). Phonological awareness skills of university students: Implications for teaching phonetics. *Contemporary Issues in Communication Sciences and Disorders, 28*, 85–90.

Nagy, W., Anderson, R. C., Schommer, M., Scott, J. A., & Stallman, A. C. (1989). Morphological families in the internal lexicon. *Reading Research Quarterly, 24*, 262–282.

Nagy, W., Berninger, V., Abbott, R., Vaughan, K., & Vermeulen, K. (2003). Relationships of morphology and other language skills to literacy skills in at-risk second-grade readers and at-risk fourth-grade writers. *Journal of Educational Psychology, 95*, 730–742.

Napps, S. E. (1989). Morphemic relationships in the lexicon: Are they distinct from semantic and formal relationships? *Memory and Cognition, 17*, 729–739.

National Center for Education Statistics. (1999). *Executive summary.* Retrieved March 22, 2004, from http://nces.ed.gov

National Institute for Literacy. (2003, June). *Put reading first: The research building blocks for teaching children to read.* Jessup, MD: Author.

Peppers, L. (1976). Patterns of leisure and adjustment to retirement. *Gerontologist, 16*, 441–446.

Qualls, C. D., & Harris, J. L. (2003). Age, working memory, figurative language type, and reading ability: Influencing factors in African American adults' comprehension of figurative language. *American Journal of Speech-Language Pathology, 12*, 92–102.

Rubin, G. S., Roche, K. B., Prasada-Rao, P., & Fried, L. P. (1994). Visual impairment and disability in older adults. *Optometry and Visual Science, 71*, 750–760.

Schuell, H. (1973). *Minnesota Test for the Differential Diagnosis of Aphasia* (2nd ed., revised by J. W. Sefer). Minneapolis: University of Minnesota Press.

Smiler, A. P., Gagne, D. D., Stine-Morrow, E. A. L. (2003). Aging, memory load, and resource allocation during reading. *Psychology and Aging, 18*, 203–109.

Smith, M. C. (1993). The reading abilities and practices of older adults. *Educational Gerontology, 19*, 417–432.

Smith, M. C. (1996). Differences in adults' reading practices and literacy proficiencies. *Reading Research Quarterly, 31*, 196–219.

Stine-Morrow, E. A. L., Loveless, M. K., & Soederberg, L. M. (1996). Resource allocation in on-line reading by younger and older adults. *Psychology and Aging, 11*, 475–486.

Stine-Morrow, E. A. L., Milinder, L., Pullara, O., & Herman, B. (2001). Patterns of resource allocation are reliable among younger and older readers. *Psychology and Aging, 16*, 69–84.

Stine-Morrow, E. A. L., Miller, L. M. S., & Leno, R. (2001). Patterns of on-line resource allocation to narrative text by younger and older adults. *Aging, Neuropsychology, and Cognition, 8*, 36–53.

Waters, G. S., & Caplan, D. (2001). Age, working memory, and on-line syntactic processing in sentence comprehension. *Psychology and Aging, 16*, 128–144.

Weiss, B., Hart, G., McGee, D., & D'Estelle, S. (1992). Health status among illiterate adults: Relation between literacy and health status among persons with low literacy skills. *Journal of the American Board of Family Medicine, 5*, 257–264.

Woodcock, R. W. (1998). *Woodcock Reading Mastery Tests–Revised.* Circle Pines, MN: American Guidance Service, Inc.

Yussen, S. R., & Glysch, R. L. (1993). Remembering stories: Studies of the limits of narrative coherence on recall. In S. R. Yussen & M. C. Smith (Eds.), *Reading across the life span* (pp. 293–321). New York: Springer-Verlag.

Zabrucky, K., & Moore, D. (1994). Contributions of working memory and evaluation and regulation of understanding adults' recall of texts. *Journal of Gerontology, 49*, 201–212.

Zelinski, E. M., & Gilewski, M. J. (1988). Memory for prose and aging: A meta-analysis. In M. L. Howe & C. J. Brainerd (Eds.), *Cognitive Development in Adulthood* (pp. 135–158). New York: Springer-Verlag.

Chapter **5**

Verbal Expression

Angela N. Burda, PhD, CCC-SLP

Introduction

Expressing ourselves verbally allows us to accomplish a great deal every day. We can wake our children for school, wish our spouse a good day, conduct a meeting at work, answer questions coworkers have about an upcoming project, inquire about the price of an item at a store, and order dinner at a restaurant. Speaking requires the integration of several activities quickly and effortlessly. For example, picture naming requires us to recognize the item, access and select the corresponding phonologic or orthographic form of the word, and then articulate the word (Nicholas, Barth, Obler, Au, & Albert, 1997). Although speech does change with age, and is frequently influenced by aspects of cognition such as working memory (Kemper & Sumner, 2001; also see Chapter 2 on cognition), these changes tend to be subtle (Mortensen, Meyer, & Humphreys, 2006). Various theoretical perspectives are documented in the literature and should be kept in mind regarding age-related changes in expression abilities (see Chapter 1 on theoretical perspectives).

This chapter will discuss aging adults' verbal expression abilities, factors that can negatively affect their verbal expression, signs that warrant referral to a speech-language pathologist or other medical professionals, and strategies that can help aging adults' verbal expression. A list of "Quick Facts" is included at the end of the chapter to summarize key points.

Older Adults' General Verbal Expression Abilities

Speech-language pathologists (SLPs) have many options to evaluate their patients' verbal abilities. Several commercially available language tests for adults divide verbal tasks into subtests (e.g., Naming, Repetition). In many cases, items are arranged in a hierarchical manner, beginning with responses that are shorter and simpler in nature and progressing to lengthier, more complex items (Bayles & Tomoeda, 1993; Helm-Estabrooks, 1992). Confrontation naming is assessed by having persons name a specific person, object, place, or action (Nicholas, Barth et al., 1997); pictures and objects are typically used. Other subtests have individuals repeat utterances and describe or define objects and pictured items (e.g., nail, comb; Bayles & Tomoeda, 1993). Verbal fluency, also referred to as generative naming, requires patients to generate items from a category within a specified period of time, such as naming as many animals as possible within one minute (Bayles & Tomoeda, 1993). Discourse samples can be obtained, typically in response to questions or while viewing action-filled pictures, such as the "Cookie Theft" picture from the *Boston Diagnostic Aphasia Examination* (Goodglass, Kaplan, & Barresi, 2001; Helm-Estabrooks, 1992; Kertesz, 2006; Schuell, 1973).

It can be difficult to obtain information about neurologically intact aging adults' verbal expression abilities. Although several research studies have explored older adults' verbal expression abilities, tasks have not necessarily mirrored those found in speech-language pathology tests. As described in Chapters 2 through 4, not all tests have included aging adults as part of the standardization process, and many have not included the ages of the normal adults in the assessment manuals (Schuell, 1973). Tests that did include normal aging adults did not necessarily make them a separate control group. Combining information from the test manuals with empirical data in the literature gives a general guide of what normal verbal expression abilities are for neurologically intact older adults.

The *Aphasia Diagnostic Profile* (ADP; Helm-Estabrooks, 1992), described in Chapter 3, includes data from 40 neurologically intact adults aged 20–99 years. While 11 of these adults fell within the age range of

60–99, the test's author did not report normative data by specific age groups. Several sections assess verbal expression in the ADP. The Fluency subtest asks patients to provide discourse samples in response to SLPs asking them questions like "Tell me exactly what happened to you" and "What can you tell me about President Kennedy?" Individuals are also asked to describe a picture depicting various activities taking place at a grocery store. Scores are recorded for "Correct Informational Units" and "Total Number of Words" for the picture description. A score for "Average Phrase Length" is obtained from the discourse task with the longest phrase lengths. Although no maximum points are possible for this subtest, normative information is available for the informational units and average phrase length. No such information is available for the total number of words. The Naming subtest is made up of 12 pictured items that "range in word frequency, number of syllables, and phonemic complexity" (Helm-Estabrooks, 1992, p. 16). Sample items include a key and a thermometer. A maximum of 36 points is possible for this subtest. The Repetition subtest has 12 utterances that also vary in word frequency, length, and complexity. Sample items include "money," "pizza," and "A terrible tornado." A maximum of 36 points is possible on this subtest. Finally, a Singing subtest asks patients to sing a familiar song associated with a picture they are shown, such as an American flag or a birthday cake. A maximum score of 9 points is possible in this subtest. With the exception of the Fluency subtest, subtests are scored using a multidimensional system that takes into account such aspects as the accuracy or the speed of the response.

The ADP's test manual reports that on the Fluency subtest, neurologically intact adults in the normative sample had an average phrase length of 14.7 words (SD = 5.2) and a mean of 21.6 information units (SD = 8.8). On the Naming subtest, they had a mean score of 35.4 (SD = 1.8) out of 36 points possible. On the Repetition subtest, healthy adults performed with a mean score of 35.9 (SD = 0.5) out of a total of 36 points. On the Singing subtest, they had a mean score of 9.0 (SD = 1.1) out of 9 possible points. Overall, neurologically intact adults ages 20–99 provided lengthy phrases and a high number of correct informational units on the Fluency subtest. They also performed with a minimum of 98% accuracy on the Naming, Repetition, and Singing subtests.

The *Arizona Battery for Communication Disorders of Dementia* (ABCD; Bayles & Tomoeda, 1993), also described in Chapters 2 through 4, included older adults (M_{age} = 70.44 years, SD = 17.07) as a separate control group. Verbal expression is assessed in the following subtests: Repetition, Object Description, Generative Naming Semantic Category, Confrontation Naming, and Concept Definition. For the Repetition subtest, patients repeat nonmeaningful phrases that are six or nine syllables in length (e.g., "Incapable top spoons"). Bayles and Tomoeda (1993) reported that older adults in their standardization sample correctly scored a mean of 67.9 (SD = 7.0) items out of a total of 75 possible items (91% correct). A group of normal young adults was also part of the standardization sample and accurately repeated with a mean score of 73.7 (SD = 2.1) items (98% correct). For the Object Description subtest, participants describe a nail as completely as possible. Although a total number of points is not given for this subtest, older adults in the normative sample provided a mean of 9.1 (SD = 2.4) descriptors of the nail, and young adults provided a mean of 10.9 (SD = 2.1) descriptors. For the Generative Naming Semantic Category subtest, persons name as many modes of transportation as they can within one minute. As with the Object Description subtest, a total number of points is not provided; however, the older adults in the test sample provided a mean of 11.4 (SD = 3.4) items, compared with the young adults who generated a mean of 13.4 (SD = 3.2) items. On the Confrontation Naming subtest, individuals name 20 pictured objects (e.g., toothbrush, stethoscope, broom). Older adults accurately named an average of 18.1 items (SD = 2.3) out of 20 possible items (91% correct). Young adults correctly named a mean of 18.6 (SD = 1.1) items (93% correct). The Concept Definition subtest has patients define pictured named items (e.g., "Give me a definition of *comb*"). Older adults scored a mean of 56.6 items correct (SD = 5.0) out of a total of 60 points (94% correct), while the young adults had a mean of 57.8 (SD = 2.9; 96% correct).

Research studies have also been conducted on older adults' verbal expression abilities. Recalling proper names is particularly difficult for aging adults (Burke, Kester Locantore, Austin, & Chae, 2004; Evrard, 2002), who reportedly find this to be their most irritating and embarrassing memory problem (Lovelace & Twohig, 1990). Although older adults may not be able to retrieve a name at a particular moment, they can usually recall it given enough time or on other occasions (Cohen & Faulkner, 1986). The greatest number of these blocks occur for the names of friends and acquaintances; however, this may reflect the greater frequency of attempts to recall these names (Cohen & Faulkner, 1986). Certain names may be easier to retrieve because they are extraordinarily descriptive (e.g., Snow White), they refer to characteristics of the person (e.g., Scrooge), or they represent a particular product (e.g., Kleenex, Xerox; Burke, Kester Locantore et al., 2004).

Despite difficulties in recalling proper names, word retrieval is not an all-or-none process (Cohen & Faulkner, 1986; Schwartz, 2002). Thus, partial information about a desired name is frequently available. Cohen and Faulkner (1986) studied older adults' recall of proper names and found that participants could often form a clear image of the target and recall known characteristics of the person, such as physical attributes, names of people encountered in the same context, and names of people similar in appearance. This information tended to be recalled more frequently than phonological features of the name, such as the first letter(s), the main vowel sound, the number of syllables, or partial matching of the sound of the name of the target. When older adults generated names that were similar to the target name, they usually recognized these as incorrect. Participants could occasionally recall the first name but not the last name or vice versa and, less frequently, recalled characteristics of the name, such as if it was old-fashioned, unusual, or foreign. Despite difficulties recalling names, aging adults can have more success in retrieving individuals' occupations or hobbies and the names of places because such information carries vivid associated imagery that may make it easier to encode and recall (Cohen & Faulkner, 1986).

Related to the recall of proper names, investigators have explored "tip-of-the-tongue" (TOT) experiences, which Brown and McNeill (1966) defined in their seminal study as the inability to recall a known word at a time when "recall is felt imminent" (p. 325). Similarly, Schwartz (2002) more recently noted, "A TOT is a strong feeling that a target word, although currently unrecallable, is known and will be recalled" (p. 5). TOT experiences increase with age and most frequently when recalling proper names and infrequently used words (Brown & Nix, 1996; Burke, MacKay, Worthley, & Wade, 1991; Cohen & Faulkner, 1986; Mortensen et al., 2006; Rastle & Burke, 1996; Schwartz, 2002). TOT experiences are often resolved by a "pop-up." This is when the target is recalled suddenly and spontaneously at a time when one is not actively engaged in retrieval attempts (Cohen & Faulkner, 1986). Resolution time for TOT experiences takes longer in older adults. Heine, Ober, and Shenaut (1999) found that adults aged 80–92 resolved almost all TOT experiences when allowed enough time to do so; however, in some cases this took several hours. Thus, when healthy older adults have TOT experiences, they have not necessarily forgotten the word, but it will likely take longer to recall (Heine et al., 1999).

Picture-naming studies have found that older adults tend to be less accurate, less fluent, and slower to respond compared with younger adults (Au, Joung, Nicholas, Obler, Kaas, & Albert, 1995; Barresi, Nicholas, Connor, Obler, & Albert, 2000; Mortensen et al., 2006). Persons in their 70s reportedly have the poorest performance (Feyereisen, 1997; Nicholas, Obler, Albert, & Goodglass, 1985) and responses that differ qualitatively compared with adults in their 60s and younger. For example, adults in their 70s and 80s tend to provide more circumlocutions than their younger counterparts (Albert, Heller, & Milberg, 1988; Hodgson & Ellis, 1998). Not surprisingly, higher-frequency names are generally retrieved faster than low-frequency names (Allen, Madden, & Crozier, 1991; Gerhard & Barry, 1999). When aged adults cannot retrieve the target word, they instead tend to produce semantic errors, circumlocutions, and word-finding comments in which they accurately discuss the category or semantic features of the word (Hodgson & Ellis, 1998; Nicholas, Obler, et al., 1985; Nickels & Howard, 1994). In addition, older adults do not tend to be verbose or off-topic when naming pictures (James, Burke, Austin, & Hulme, 1998), possibly because it is a fairly easy, highly constrained task (Arbuckle, Nohara-LeClair, & Pushkar, 2000).

Some investigators have used the Boston Naming Test (BNT; Kaplan, Goodglass, & Weintraub, 1983) to measure older adults' naming abilities. The BNT is made up of 60 line drawings of objects that vary in familiarity (e.g., bed, abacus). A study by Nicholas, Barth, and colleagues (1997) reported that aging adults exhibit a wider range of performance on the BNT compared with younger adults. Connor, Spiro, Obler, and Albert (2004) measured adults' performance on the BNT over 20 years. Participants were divided into the following age groups: 30–39, 50–59, 60–69, and 70–80 years. If persons could not name an item (e.g., accordion) because of difficulty recognizing the picture (e.g., "It's a high-rise building"), a semantic cue was given (e.g., "It's a musical instrument"). If the response was incorrect but semantically related (e.g., "piano"), an eliciting cue was provided (e.g., "Is there another word for that?"). If individuals still could not respond or their answer was incorrect, a phonemic cue was supplied (e.g., "acc-"). The investigators found that older adults' performance declined an average of two percentage points per decade. Although there was a slight acceleration as individuals got older, the decline was subtle with many individual differences in the rate of change. Also, while those in the 60 to 69 and 70–79 groups received the most phonemic cues, all age groups benefited equally from these cues.

Mayr and Kliegl (2000) measured verbal fluency in older adults (M_{age} = 69 years) and younger adults (M_{age} = 24 years). Semantic categories of varying difficulty were used. Examples of easy categories included clothes, foods, and four-legged animals. Categories classified as a medium level of difficulty included kitchen utensils, fish, and weather phenomena. Samples of difficult categories were fabrics, traffic signs, and insects. The authors found that errors were generally rare. When errors did occur, they were most frequently within category perseverations (e.g., saying "dog" twice for four-legged animals), but even older adults rarely exhibited perseverations. Older participants did run out of time significantly more often than the young adults, typically toward the end of the recall sequences for the difficult categories.

Repetition abilities have been investigated in the aged. Kemper (1986) had older adults (70–89 years) and younger adults (30–49 years) repeat grammatical and ungrammatical complex sentences with embedded clauses. Sentences represented four topics: baking cookies, working in a hardware store, watching the Olympics, and growing flowers. Sentences varied in grammatical correctness, length of the embedded clauses, position of the embedded clause (beginning or end of sentence), and the type of embedded clause. The four types of embedded clauses used were: gerunds ("Baking tires me out"), wh-clauses ("What I did interested my grandchildren"), that-clauses ("That the cookies were brown surprised me"), and relative clauses ("My grandchildren enjoyed the cookies I baked"). Participants could correct any sentence they judged to be ungrammatical. Both groups generally produced grammatical repetitions for sentences with short embedded clauses. Although older adults corrected ungrammatical sentences, they made more errors than the young adults. They were also unable to repeat or paraphrase long constructions, especially when embedded clauses were found in the beginning of the sentence and when these sentences were ungrammatical (e.g., "Baking ginger cookies for my grandchildren am tires me out"). In such instances, aging adults typically responded with ungrammatical sentences, evaluative judgments, or personal associations. In general, older adults can accurately imitate or paraphrase short sentences but have marked difficulty repeating and paraphrasing lengthy, complex syntactic structures.

Discourse abilities in the aging population have been widely studied using various tasks to elicit speech samples. In studies in which participants describe pictures, such as the "Cookie Theft" picture from the *Boston Diagnostic Aphasia Examination* (Goodglass & Kaplan, 1983), older adults used more indefinite words such as "thing" (Cooper, 1990; Obler, 1980). Two more recent studies have also employed pictures to measure older adults' discourse. Juncos-Rabadán, Pereiro, and Soledad Rodríguez (2005) had differently aged adults tell stories when viewing cartoon strips depicting different activities (e.g., walking a dog, burning dinner). Although aging adults expressed the same amount of content in the stories compared with middle-aged adults, they used more words, had a lower percentage of pronouns with a clear reference, and had more irrelevant speech. In another study, Marini, Boewe, Caltagirone, and Carlomagno (2005) had participants ages 20–84 describe the "Picnic" picture from the *Western Aphasia Battery* (Kertesz, 1982) and two cartoon sequences. The oldest group (75–84) had the greatest variation in performance, produced more paraphasias and tangential speech, had sharp drops in syntactic complexity, and had difficulty relating utterances to each other (Marini et al., 2005). Although informativeness gradually decreased with age, all age groups produced narratives that generally focused on the main themes of the pictures. Also, the ratio of main ideas to details was 1:1 in the oldest groups. The authors hypothesized that older persons may get better at constructing themes and emphasizing relevant details, thus providing more effective descriptions and stories. Interestingly, speech characteristics that are usually considered pathologic were present in the healthy older adults, including paragrammatisms, semantic paraphasias, and ambiguous referencing.

Some investigators have used autobiographical interviews in their discourse research. James and colleagues (1998) found that older adults had significantly more words and off-topic speech when producing autobiographical narratives, but their samples were rated more interesting and informative than those of young adults. Some of this verbosity may be attributed to aging adults having different communication goals. In particular, they tend to emphasize the descriptions of their personal experiences over reporting facts (James et al., 1998). More recently, Kemper, Marquis, and Thompson (2001) elicited autobiographical narratives over the course of 7–17 years from adults who were ages 65–75 at the first assessment and ages 79–83 at the final assessment. Sample questions included "Describe the persons who most influenced your life" and "Describe an unexpected event that happened to you." Measures were taken on propositional density and grammatical complexity. Propositional density refers to how much information is conveyed relative to the number of words spoken (Kemper & Sumner, 2001). The most pronounced declines in grammatical complexity and propositional density (i.e., using more words to convey a message) occurred between the ages of 74 and 78, with more gradual declines before and after that interval. However, there was considerable individual variation in older adults' initial levels of grammatical complexity and propositional density as well as in their levels of decline.

Procedural discourse has also been investigated. North, Ulatowska, Malacuso-Haynes, and Bell (1986) had a group of older women (M_{age} = 76.2 years) and a group of middle-aged women (M_{age} = 45.6 years) perform three procedural-discourse tasks. Specifically, participants were asked to describe all of the steps involved in mailing a letter, polishing shoes, and shopping at a nearby store. Both age groups accurately sequenced the steps in each task, although the older women did not provide as many steps as the middle-aged women (North et al., 1986).

Language analyses show that older adults tend to favor producing right-branching constructions of sentences over left-branching constructs. In left-branching constructions (e.g., "*The gal who runs a nursery school for our church* is awfully young"), the embedded clause occurs to the left of the main clause. Thus, the subject "the gal" must be retained and the main clause "is" must be anticipated as the embedded clause "who runs a nursery school for our church" is being produced. In right-branching sentences (e.g., "She's awfully young *to be running a nursery for our church*"), each clause is produced sequentially and the embedded clause occurs to the right of the main clause (Kemper, Marquis, & Thompson, 2001). Asymmetry between left- and right-branching constructions may reflect declines in working memory (Gibson, 1988).

In Burda's 2007 study, described in Chapter 3, 31 adults aged 65 and older were divided into three age categories: Young-Old (M_{age} = 69.3 years), Middle-Old (M_{age} = 81.1 years), and Old-Old (M_{age} = 89.5 years).

Participants performed various verbal-expression tasks, including: naming pictures (e.g., mirror, pen) and objects (e.g., whistle, spoon), and completing responsive-naming tasks in which they named the object described by its function (e.g., "You shine it in the dark" for "flashlight"). Individuals also completed divergent-categorization tasks in which they provided five items in a given category (e.g., words that begin with the letter *s*, things that are cold). Ten categories were used. The categories selected were considered to be more complex in nature versus more concrete (e.g., foods, animals). Participants were allotted as much time as needed to complete all tasks. Items for the naming and description tasks were selected from the *Language Activities Resource Kit*, 2nd edition (Dressler, 2001). Divergent-categorization tasks were chosen from *Speech and Language Rehabilitation*, 4th edition (Keith & Schumacher, 2000). Results are included in **Table 5-1**, broken down by age groups.

As shown in Table 5-1, participants had high accuracy levels for all of the tasks. No marked differences occurred across the age groups, and no statistically significant differences occurred in performance among the three age groups. It should be noted the sample size for this pilot study was small.

In summary, based on information included in the normative data for adult language tests and in research studies, older adults should be able to complete confrontational naming, responsive naming, repetition, object description, divergent categorization, and singing tasks with a minimum of 90% accuracy. Despite the high accuracy rates for these various tasks, older adults' naming abilities tend to be less accurate, less fluent, and slower compared with those of young adults, and their performance on the BNT (Kaplan et al., 1983) declines an average of two percentage points per decade. Aging adults will likely experience difficulty recalling names and have more TOT experiences;

Table 5-1

Mean Performance for Verbal-Expression Tasks

Task	Total*	Young-Old			Middle-Old			Old-Old		
		M	*SD*	%**	*M*	*SD*	%**	*M*	*SD*	%**
Picture naming	10	10.0	0.0	100	9.7	0.6	97	9.8	0.4	98
Object naming	10	10.0	0.0	100	10.0	0.0	100	10.0	0.0	100
Responsive naming	10	9.9	0.3	99	10.0	0.0	100	9.7	0.5	97
Divergent categorization	50	49.8	0.4	99	49.4	0.8	99	49.2	1.4	98

Note: *refers to the total number of points possible. **refers to the percentage correct.
Source: Burda (2007).

however, they can usually recall the desired name or word given enough time, which in some cases may be several hours. For verbal-fluency tasks, aging adults should be able to generate an average of 11 items in a given category, typically without any errors; however, they are more likely to run out of time if a category is difficult. If they do produce errors, these tend to be repetitions of prior responses. Older adults can accurately repeat or paraphrase short sentences but have difficulty with lengthy, syntactically complex utterances.

In general, discourse studies report that older adults use more words and produce more irrelevant speech to express an idea than younger adults. They are more disfluent when tasks are difficult, such as when conversing about unfamiliar topics or when few constraints are placed on the content of the utterances. They also get off-topic more easily during conversational speech. However, aging adults are not as disfluent or verbose when discussing familiar topics, and they can adequately complete procedural-discourse tasks, although they may provide fewer steps in a sequence. Healthy adults ages 65–80 evidence reduced linguistic abilities, including producing fewer grammatical forms, syntactic structures, and verb tenses. The most rapid declines in propositional density and grammatical complexity occur in the mid-70s. In addition, adults in their 70s and 80s tend to have less complex responses than 50- and 60-year-olds. Older adults can display more word-retrieval difficulty during discourse. They produce more filler words (e.g., "Well, you know"), non-lexical fillers (e.g., "uh," "um"), and repeated words, which may mask word-retrieval problems and allow time to find the target words. They also produce speech characteristics typically considered pathological, such as paragrammatisms, semantic paraphasias, and ambiguous referencing. Despite age-related speech differences, several positive trends are reported. Older adults can have larger vocabularies than younger adults (see Verhaegen, 2003); most of their linguistic skills remain preserved across the life span or decline very gradually; their conversational abilities are usually well preserved; and the presence of linguistic anomalies does not make their speech unintelligible (Marini et al., 2005, Shadden, 1997). Healthy older adults may be able to do far more than is reported here, and more research is needed to further document their abilities.

Factors Affecting Older Adults' Verbal Expressions and Signs of Problems

Cognitive functioning can affect older adults' verbal expression. Declines in linguistic abilities between the ages of 65 and 80 are partially attributed to working memory limitations (Kemper, Marquis, & Thompson, 2001). Reduced working memory and attention can lead to difficulty recalling words and names (Cohen & Burke, 1993) and to speech that is syntactically less complex and more verbose (Kemper, 1986; Kemper & Sumner, 2001; Kemper, Marquis, & Thompson, 2001; Kynette & Kemper, 1986; Marini et al., 2005). Verbal tasks that have time constraints or demand a great deal of cognitive resources, such as spontaneously producing or repeating lengthy complex utterances or discussing unfamiliar topics, can lead to speech that is slower, more verbose, and/or more disfluent (Bortfeld, Leon, Bloom, Schober, & Brennan, 2001; Kemper, Herman, & Lian, 2003; Spieler & Griffin, 2006). When producing oral autobiographies, healthy older adults with higher scores on the Mini-Mental State Examination (MMSE; Folstein, Folstein, & McHugh, 1975) have less-varied vocabulary, longer utterances, more clauses per utterances, and fewer fragments than that of persons with lower MMSE scores who generate shorter, simpler sentences and more fragments (Mitzner & Kemper, 2003). In addition, those who have higher digit span scores (i.e., repeating strings of numbers) are likely to have increased grammatical complexity, however, this ability can decline more rapidly compared with older adults who have lower digit span scores (Kemper, Marquis, & Thompson, 2001). Similarly, healthy aging adults with higher vocabulary scores tend to display higher propositional density but show more rapid declines in this ability than those with lower vocabulary scores (Kemper, Marquis, & Thompson, 2001). However, Connor and colleagues (2004) report that persons with initially higher performance on the BNT (Kaplan et al., 1983) show less declines over time, possibly indicating that persons who have some combination of high levels of intelligence, education, and a cognitively active lifestyle have more brain reserve or are better able to compensate for changes in performance. Processing efficiency also diminishes with age, making it more challenging for older adults to rapidly access and retrieve information (e.g., target word) from long-term memory (Kemper & Sumner, 2001).

Health, physical condition, educational level, and the age when words are acquired also factor into older adults' verbal expression abilities. As previously reported, persons in their 70s evidence less complex sentences but use more words to convey their message. These changes may correspond to declining health (Kemper, Marquis, & Thompson, 2001; Small & Backman, 1999). Aging adults in better physical condition tend to produce more right-branching clauses, more clauses per utterance, longer utterances, and more grammatically complex utterances than those in poorer physical condition (Mitzner & Kemper, 2003). When older adults are feeling tired, stressed, or unwell, they demonstrate increases in the incidence and severity in the inability to recall names (Cohen & Faulkner, 1986). While educational level appears to have little effect on the accurate repetition of sentences (Kemper, 1986) or when producing oral autobiographies

(Mitzner & Kemper, 2003), older adults with lower educational levels demonstrate poorer naming abilities (Connor et al., 2004; Neils, Baris, Carter, Dell'aira, Nordloh, Weiler, & Weisiger, 1995). Older adults' naming abilities can also be affected by the age at which individuals acquire the names of objects (Gerhard & Barry, 1999; Hodgson & Ellis, 1998). Age of acquisition refers to when words are learned versus how long they have resided in memory (Hodgson & Ellis, 1998). Poon and Fozard (1978) had older and younger adults name items that were considered unique aged objects (e.g., bedpan), unique contemporary objects (e.g., calculator), common aged objects (e.g., old telephone), and common contemporary objects (e.g., modern phone). Older adults named the aged objects faster than the contemporary objects, while young adults named the contemporary objects more quickly than the aged objects. Finally, one theory is that older adults display increased verbosity because they are more isolated than younger adults; however, research studies do not support this hypothesis (Mortensen et al., 2006).

Several signs can indicate if older adults are having difficulty with verbal expression and should be referred to a speech-language pathologist (SLP) and/or other medical professionals. If older adults complain about their speech or notice a change in their ability to communicate verbally, they should be seen by their physician and an SLP. A sudden onset of slurred speech can be a sign of a stroke or transient ischemic attack (TIA; Al-Wabil, Smith, Moyé, Burgin, & Morgenstern, 2003). A TIA is sometimes referred to as a mini-stroke because symptoms typically resolve within 24 hours of onset. If sudden onset of slurred speech occurs, family members or caregivers should immediately call 911, as time is of the essence in treating strokes (Zerwic, Young Hwang, & Tucco, 2007).

Other signs of problems with verbal expression include word-finding difficulties. While some degree of word-retrieval difficulty can be normal in healthy aging adults, such difficulty may also be a sign of neurological problems, particularly if it persists and worsens over time. Older individuals who frequently repeat previously stated information should also be seen by SLPs and their physicians. As with word-retrieval difficulties, aging adults may occasionally repeat certain stories or events; however, frequent repetition may be a sign of underlying neurological problems. Changes in older individuals' grammatical complexity may be signs of cognitive disorders, although even those with dementia can still produce grammatical sentences and can convey a great deal despite word-finding and memory problems (Kemper, Marquis, & Thompson, 2001). In addition, healthy older adults tend to have age-related declines in their syntactic complexity. Nevertheless, it is still appropriate to have aging adults see their physicians and SLPs in order to determine if verbal expression changes are simply a result of aging or are due to neurological impairments. Older individuals who have difficulties with verbal expression may withdraw from social activities and other endeavors that they previously enjoyed. Lack of involvement in previously enjoyed activities can also be a sign of depression (Markowitz, 2008), warranting a thorough medical evaluation. If any of these signs occur, aging adults would benefit from being seen by the appropriate medical professionals.

Strategies to Help Older Adults' Verbal Expression

Several strategies can assist older adults' verbal expression. The majority focus on aiding name and word retrieval. Tactics they can try include: using circumlocution and synonyms, mentally running through the alphabet, generating names from a single context (e.g., names of all neighbors), reliving past experiences to enhance the description of the person, looking up the name, or asking someone else to supply the word (Cohen & Faulkner, 1986; Heine et al., 1999). Creating a mental image that relates to a specific word or a name can link the meaning of the word with an interactive image (Begg, 1983; Einstein & McDaniel, 2004). Examples include associating the name of "Gordon" with the image of a garden (Cohen & Faulkner, 1986) or associating the street name of "Edgemont" with an image of a person standing on the edge of a mountain. Practice saying the desired word to be remembered can be helpful (Connor et al., 2004) because its production helps strengthen connections in the brain and facilitates subsequent productions (Rastle & Burke, 1996). When TOT experiences occur, older adults should be allowed as much time as needed to recall the target word because they frequently have an automatic resolution (i.e., "pop-up"; Heine et al., 1999). Relatedly, allowing as much time as needed to speak leads to more fluent and more accurate speech (Spieler & Griffin, 2006).

Research has been done on older adults' naming abilities when primes and cues are given. A prime refers to a spoken or written word that precedes the item that is to be named (Mortensen et al., 2006). Cues, in contrast, are provided after persons try to retrieve a word. Older adults do benefit from phonological priming (Mortensen et al., 2006) as well as from several types of cues. Examples include phonological cues (e.g., first sound of the word), orthographic cues (e.g., first written letter of word followed by dashes representing the remaining letters of the word), and semantic cues (e.g., a related word; Bowles & Poon, 1985; Gruneberg & Monks, 1974; Heine et al., 1999; Woo & Schmitter-Edgecombe, 2009). Such strategies may not be practical because they could embarrass older adults and because communication partners might not know what their aging counterparts want to say. However, conversation partners may be able to ask helpful questions if older adults are unable to retrieve a word or name (e.g., "Is it one of your golfing partners?").

Quick Facts

- General Verbal Expression Abilities of Neurologically Intact Older Adults:
  - Can complete confrontational naming, responsive naming, repetition, object description, divergent categorization, and singing tasks generally with a minimum of 90% accuracy
  - Have naming abilities that are less accurate, less fluent, and slower than that of young adults
  - Experience performance declines on the Boston Naming Test an average of two percentage points per decade
  - Experience difficulty recalling words and names and have more TOT experiences
  - Generate an average of 11 items in verbal-fluency tasks
  - Accurately repeat and paraphrase short sentences but have difficulty with lengthy, complex utterances
  - Use more words, produce more irrelevant speech, and get off-topic during discourse
  - Are more disfluent when discussing unfamiliar topics
  - Adequately complete procedural-discourse tasks, although they may provide fewer steps in a sequence
  - Produce fewer grammatical forms, syntactic structures, and verb tenses with most rapid declines in propositional density and grammatical complexity during their 70s
  - Produce items typically considered pathological: paragrammatisms, semantic paraphasias, and ambiguous referencing
  - Positive trends include:
    - Older adults can have larger vocabularies than younger adults
    - Most linguistic skills remain preserved across life span or decline only gradually
    - Presence of linguistic anomalies does not make speech unintelligible
- Factors That Can Negatively Affect Older Adults' Verbal Expression:
  - Reduced working memory, attention, and processing efficiency
  - Verbal tasks that have time constraints or demand a great deal of cognitive resources, such as spontaneously producing or repeating lengthy complex utterances or discussing unfamiliar topics

- Declining health, poor physical condition, or feeling tired, stressed, or unwell
- Lower education level
- Age at which the names of items are acquired
- Signs That an Older Adult Should Be Referred to a Speech-Language Pathologist or Other Medical Professionals:
  - Overt complaints of difficulty or changes in their speech
  - A sudden onset of slurred speech. Get medical help immediately (e.g., dial 9-1-1)
  - Word-finding difficulties
  - Frequent repetition of previously stated information
  - Changes in the grammatical complexity of speech
  - Withdrawing from social activities or other activities previously enjoyed
- Strategies That Can Help Older Adults' Verbal Expression:
  - Encourage use of circumlocutions and synonyms during word-retrieval difficulties
  - Give older adults strategies to recall words and names:
    - Run through the alphabet
    - Generate names from a single context (e.g., name all neighbors)
    - Relive past experiences to enhance the description of the person
    - Look up the name
    - Ask someone to supply the word
    - Create a mental image that can be associated with a specific word or name
  - Allow as much time as needed to recall target words and to speak in general
  - Encourage older adults to practice saying the target word
  - Ask questions if word-retrieval difficulties occur

Discussion Questions

1. Are there any theories that address why older adults have different communication objectives than younger adults?
2. How does the mental well-being (e.g., presence of stress or depression) of older adults affect their verbal expression?
3. How do the topics that individuals like to discuss change as they age?
4. Older adults' narrative samples are reportedly more interesting. What kinds of examples do you have from your own life in which you found this to be true?

References

Al-Wabil, A., Smith, M. A., Moyé, L. A., Burgin, W. S., & Morgenstern, L. B. (2003). Improving efficiency of stroke research: The Brain Attack Surveillance in Corpus Christi study. *Journal of Clinical Epidemiology, 56*, 351–357.

Albert, M. S., Heller, H. S., & Milberg, W. (1988). Changes in naming ability with age. *Psychology Aging, 3*, 173–178.

Allen, P. A., Madden, D. J., & Crozier, L. C. (1991). Adult age differences in letter-level and word-level processing. *Psychology and Aging, 6*, 261–271.

Arbuckle, T. Y., Nohara-LeClair, M., & Pushkar, D. (2000). Effect of off-target verbosity on communication efficiency in a referential communication task. *Psychology and Aging, 15*, 65–77.

Au, R., Joung, P., Nicholas, M., Obler, L., Kass, R., & Albert, M. L. (1995). Naming ability across the adult life span. *Aging and Cognition, 2*, 302–311.

Barresi, B. A., Nicholas, M., Connor, L. T., Obler, L. K., & Albert, M. L. (2000). Semantic degradation and lexical access in age-related naming failures. *Aging, Neuropsychology, and Cognition, 7*, 169–178.

Bayles, K. A., & Tomoeda, C. K. (1993). *Arizona Battery for Communication Disorders of Dementia.* Tucson, AZ: Canyonlands Publishing.

Begg, I. (1983). Imagery instructions and the organization of memory. In J. C. Yuille (Ed.), *Imagery, memory, and cognition: Essays in honor of Allan Paivio* (pp. 91–115). Hillsdale, NJ: Erlbaum.

Bortfeld, H., Leon, S. D., Bloom, J. E., Schober, M. F., & Brennan, S. E. (2001). Disfluency rates in conversation: Effects of age, relationship, topic, role, and gender. *Language and Speech, 44*, 123–147.

Bowles, N. L., & Poon, L. W. (1985). Aging and retrieval of words in semantic memory. *Journal of Gerontology, 40*, 71–77.

Brown, A. S., & Nix, L. A. (1996). Age-related changes in the tip-of-the-tongue experience. *American Journal of Psychology, 109*, 79–91.

Brown, R., & McNeill, D. (1966). The "tip-of-the-tongue" phenomenon. *Journal of Verbal Learning and Verbal Behavior, 5*, 325–337.

Burda, A. N. (2007). *Communication changes in healthy aging adults.* Adele Whitenack Davis Research in Gerontology Award, University of Northern Iowa.

Burke, D. M., Kester Locantore, J., Austin, A. A., & Chae, B. (2004). Cherry pit primes Brad Pitt: Homophone priming effects on young and older adults' production of proper names. *Psychological Science, 15*, 164–170.

Burke, D. M., MacKay, D. G., Worthley, J. S., & Wade, E. (1991). On the tip of the tongue: What causes word finding failures in young and older adults? *Journal of Memory and Language, 30*, 542–579.

Cohen, G., & Burke, D. M. (1993). Memory for proper names: A review. *Memory, 1*, 249–263.

Cohen, G., & Faulkner, D. (1986). Does "elderspeak" work? The effect of intonation and stress on comprehension and recall of spoken discourse in old age. *Language and Communication, 6*, 91–98.

Connor, L. T., Spiro, A., III, Obler, L. K., & Albert, M. L. (2004). Change in object naming ability during adulthood. *Journal of Gerontology: Psychological Sciences, 59B*, P203–P209.

Cooper, P. V. (1990). Discourse production and normal aging performance on oral picture description tasks. *Journal of Gerontology: Psychological Sciences, 45*, 210–214.

Dressler, R. A. (2001). *Language Activities Resource Kit* (2nd ed.). Dedham, MA: AliMed.

Einstein, G. O., & McDaniel, M. A. (2004). Memory fitness: A guide for successful aging. New Haven, CT: Yale University Press.

Evrard, M. (2002). Ageing and lexical access to common and proper names in picture naming. Brain and Language, 81, 174–179.

Feyereisen, P. (1997). A meta-analytic procedure shows an age-related decline in picture naming. Journal of Speech, Language, and Hearing Research, 40, 1328–1333.

Folstein, M. F., Folstein, S. E., & McHugh, P. R. (1975). Mini-Mental State: A practical method for grading the cognitive state of patients for the clinician. Journal of Psychiatric Research, 12, 189–198.

Gerhard, S., & Barry, C. (1999). Age of acquisition, word frequency, and the role of phonology in the lexical decision task. Memory and Cognition, 27, 592–602.

Gibson, E. (1988). Syntactic complexity: Locality of syntactic dependencies. Cognition, 68, 1–76.

Goodglass, H., & Kaplan, E. (1983). The Boston Diagnostic Aphasia Examination. Philadelphia: Lea & Febiger.

Goodglass, H., Kaplan, E., & Barresi, B. (2001). Boston Diagnostic Aphasia Examination (3rd ed.). Philadelphia: Lippincott Williams & Wilkins.

Gruneberg, M. M., & Monks, J. (1974). "Feeling of knowing" and cued recall. Acta Psychologica, 38, 257–265.

Heine, M. K., Ober, B. A., & Shenaut, G. K. (1999). Naturally occurring and experimentally induced tip-of-the-tongue experiences in three adult age groups. Psychology and Aging, 14, 445–457.

Helm-Estabrooks, N. (1992). Aphasia Diagnostic Profile. Dedham, MA: AliMed.

Hodgson, C., & Ellis, A. W. (1998). Last in, first to go: Age of acquisition and naming in the elderly. Brain and Language, 64, 146–163.

James, L. E., Burke, D. M., Austin, A. & Hulme, E. (1998). Production and perception of "verbosity" in younger and older adults. Psychological Aging, 13, 355–367.

Juncos-Rabadán, O., Pereiro, A. X., & Soledad Rodríguez, M. (2005). Narrative speech in aging: Quantity, information content, and cohesion. Brain and Language, 95, 423–434.

Kaplan, E. F., Goodglass, H., & Weintraub, S. (1983). The Boston Naming Test (2nd ed.). Philadelphia: Lea & Febiger.

Keith, R. L., & Schumacher, J. G. (2000). Speech and Language Rehabilitation (4th ed.). Austin, TX: Pro-Ed.

Kemper, S. (1986). Imitation of complex syntactic constructions by elderly adults. Applied Psycholinguistics, 7, 277–288.

Kemper, S., Herman, R. E., & Lian, C. H. (2003). The costs of doing two things at once for young and older adults: Talking while walking, finger tapping, and ignoring speech or noise. Psychology and Aging, 18, 181–192.

Kemper, S., Marquis, J., & Thompson, M. (2001). Longitudinal changes in language production: Effects of aging and dementia on grammatical complexity and propositional content. Psychology and Aging, 16, 600–614.

Kemper, S., & Sumner, A. (2001). The structure of verbal abilities in young and older adults. Psychology and Aging, 16, 312–322.

Kertesz, A. (1982). Western Aphasia Battery. New York: Grune & Stratton.

Kertesz, A. (2006). Western Aphasia Battery–Revised. San Antonio, TX: Harcourt Assessment, Inc.

Kynette, D., & Kemper, S. (1986). Aging and the loss of grammatical forms: A cross-sectional study of language performance. Language and Communication, 6, 65–72.

Lovelace, E. A., & Twohig, P. T. (1990). Healthy older adults' perceptions of their memory functioning and use of mnemonics. Bulletin of the Psychonomic Society, 28, 115–118.

Marini, A., Boewe, A., Caltagirone, C., & Carlomagno, S. (2005). Age-related differences in the production of textual descriptions. *Journal of Psycholinguistic Research, 34*, 439–463.

Markowitz, J. (2008). Evidence-based psychotherapies for depression. *Journal of Occupational and Environmental Medicine, 50*, 437–440.

Mayr, U., & Kliegl, R. (2000). Complex semantic processing in old age: Does it stay or does it go? *Psychology and Aging, 15*, 29–43.

Mitzner, T. L., & Kemper, S. (2003). Oral and written language in late adulthood: Findings from the Nun Study. *Experimental Aging Research, 29*, 457–474.

Mortensen, L., Meyer, A. S., & Humphreys, G. W. (2006). Age-related effects on speech production: A review. *Language and Cognitive Processes, 21*, 238–290.

Neils, J., Baris, J. M., Carter, C., Dell'aira, A. L., Nordloh, S. J., Weiler, E., & Weisiger, B. (1995). Effects of age, education, and living environment on Boston Naming Test performance. *Journal of Speech and Hearing Research, 38*, 1143–1149.

Nicholas, M., Barth, C., Obler, L. K., Au, R., & Albert, M. L. (1997). Naming in normal aging and dementia of the Alzheimer's type. In H. Goodglass & A. Wingfield (Eds.), *Anomia: Neuroanatomical and cognitive correlates.* (pp. 166–188). San Diego, CA: Academic Press.

Nicholas, M., Obler, L., Albert, M., & Goodglass, H. (1985). Lexical retrieval in healthy aging. *Cortex, 21*, 595–606.

Nickels, L., & Howard, D. (1994). A frequent occurrence? Factors affecting the production of semantic errors in aphasic naming. *Cognitive Neuropsychology, 11*, 289–320.

North, A. J., Ulatowska, H. K., Macaluso-Haynes, S., & Bell, H. (1986). Discourse performance in older adults. *International Journal of Aging and Human Development, 23*, 267–283.

Obler, L. K. (1980). Narrative discourse style in the elderly. In L. K. Obler & M. L. Albert (Eds.), *Language and communication in the elderly* (pp. 75–90). Lexington, MA: D. C. Health.

Poon, L. W., & Fozard, J. L. (1978). Speed of retrieval from long-term memory in relation to age, familiarity, and datedness of information. *Journal of Gerontology, 33*, 711–717.

Rastle, K. G., & Burke, D. M. (1996). Priming the tip of the tongue: Effects of prior processing on word retrieval in young and older adults. *Journal of Memory and Language, 35*, 586–605.

Schuell, H. (1973). *Minnesota Test for the Differential Diagnosis of Aphasia* (2nd ed., revised by J. W. Sefer). Minneapolis: University of Minnesota Press.

Schwartz, B. L. (2002). *Tip-of-the-tongue states: Phenomenology, mechanism, and lexical retrieval.* Mahwah, NJ: Lawrence Erlbaum Associates.

Shadden, B. B. (1997). Discourse behaviors in older adults. *Seminars in Speech and Language, 18*, 143–156.

Small, B. J., & Backman, L. (1999). Time to death and cognitive performance. *Current Directions in Psychological Sciences, 8*, 168–172.

Spieler, D. H., & Griffin, Z. M. (2006). The influence of age on the time course of word preparation in multiword utterances. *Language and Cognitive Processes, 21*, 291–321.

Verhaegen, P. (2003). Aging and vocabulary scores: A meta-analysis. *Psychology and Aging, 18*, 332–339.

Woo, E., & Schmitter-Edgecombe, M. (2009). Aging and semantic cueing during learning and retention verbal episodic information. *Aging, Neuropsychology, and Cognition, 16*, 103–119.

Zerwic, J., Young Hwang, S., & Tucco, L. (2007). Interpretation of symptoms and delay in seeking treatment by patients who have had a stroke: Exploratory study. *Heart and Lung, 36*, 25–34.

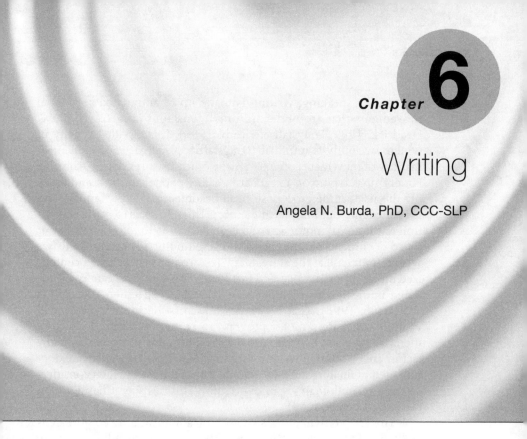

Chapter **6**

Writing

Angela N. Burda, PhD, CCC-SLP

Introduction

Whether it is signing our names to legal documents, writing a grocery list, or typing an e-mail, most people are able to communicate through the written word. Despite the relative efficiency of writing (Alamargot & Chanquoy, 2001), it is actually a complex psychomotor activity (Andersen, 1969; Longstaff & Heath, 1997) that reflects how people think, feel, and behave (Wellingham-Jones, 1989). Writing can be revised to better reflect what individuals wish to convey (Tynjälä, Mason, & Lonka, 2001) and can be changed according to its purpose (Mitzner & Kemper, 2003). For example, writers may take more care and have significantly different content when writing a thank-you note to a family member than when quickly jotting down a to-do list at the start of a work day.

Writing is unique in that it requires adequate cognitive-linguistic and motor abilities. Individuals must possess generally intact semantic, syntactic, lexical, and phonological systems (Graham & Weintraub, 1996) and sufficient memory abilities (Hoskyn & Swanson, 2003).

Motorically speaking, writing is made up of automated sequential movements that are under minimal conscious control (Huber & Headrick, 1999; Longstaff & Heath, 1997). It is a skilled activity in which variability is minimal (Longstaff & Heath, 1997). Such automaticity of movements occurs in many other instances during daily life. For example, typing on a keyboard, dialing phone numbers, and walking the aisles at the grocery store all become motorically familiar and ingrained into our long-term memory. This allows us to pay less attention to the actual motor acts and more attention to the content of our typed documents and phone calls or the finding of specific items we wish to purchase at the store. Many researchers believe that a centralized motor program exists and that lower-level processes cannot be initiated until higher-order processes have been specified (Graham & Weintraub, 1996). That is, writers must first decide what they will write in order for a motor program to be retrieved from long-term memory (Graham & Weintraub, 1996). Thus, it is apparent that many factors are involved in writing. Various theoretical perspectives are documented in the literature and should be kept in mind when considering age-related changes in expression abilities (see Chapter 1 on theoretical perspectives).

This chapter will discuss what aging adults' writing abilities generally should be, factors that can negatively affect older adults' writing, signs that may warrant referral to a speech-language pathologist or other medical professionals, and what strategies can help aging adults write. A list of "Quick Facts" at the end of the chapter summarizes important points.

Older Adults' General Writing Abilities

When individuals are evaluated by speech-language pathologists (SLPs), their writing abilities are one of many areas that are systematically assessed. Handwriting can be a somewhat challenging area to evaluate because SLPs must look not only at the accuracy of the content but also how legible and grammatically correct the sample is. Legibility refers to the readability of a handwriting sample and can include features such as size, slant, spacing, and uniformity of one's writing (Andersen, 1969; Rubin & Henderson, 1982; Tomchek & Schneck, 2005). It can be difficult to discern the content if the legibility is poor. SLPs note whether misspellings are evident or if a lack of punctuation occurs. They also pay attention to whether or not letters are misshapen or if the spacing is inconsistent. Because writing can differ based on the hand used (Wright, 1990), clinicians want to know the dominant hand that individuals use when writing, and if that differs from the hand utilized during the evaluation. This is crucial because writing may not be as fluent or the letters may not be as accurately shaped when the non-dominant hand is used (Kopeenhaver, 2007; Wright, 1990). It is important to know what kind of writing individuals have done over the course of their lives, particularly in more recent times. It is also imperative for SLPs to know if individuals struggled with writing at any point in their lives, if they consider themselves "good writers" or "bad writers," and if they are required to write as part of their daily routines. Some individuals have always had significant difficulty with writing, and in their current living situation, they may do very little writing. All of these factors can impact SLPs' decisions when selecting areas to address in therapy. Of significant importance are older adults' abilities to write and sign their names as well as write biographical information (e.g., address, birthdate; Helm-Estabrooks, 1992). Such information is frequently requested on various medical, financial, and legal documents (Walton, 1997), making these necessary abilities to evaluate. In commercially available language and cognition tests for adults, writing tasks generally include providing biographical information (as previously indicated), writing letters and numbers, copying and drawing figures or geometric shapes, writing words and/or sentences to dictation, writing spontaneous sentences, and writing paragraphs (e.g., after viewing a picture; Bayles & Tomoeda, 1993; Helm-Estabrooks, 1992, 2001; Kertesz, 2006; Schuell, 1973).

Information about neurologically intact aging adults' writing abilities can be challenging to find. Research studies have not necessarily included clinical tasks found in speech-language pathology tests, such as those previously mentioned (e.g., biographical information). As previously described, all tests have not systematically included aging adults as part of the standardization process or have not included the ages of the normal adults in the assessment manuals (Schuell, 1973). In certain cases, the normal group could be considered questionable. For example, as described in Chapter 3, prisoners solely compose the group of normal adults included in the *Aphasia Language Performance Scale* (ALPS; Keenan & Brassell, 1975). Some exceptions exist, and information found in test manuals coupled with empirical data in the literature can provide a general guide on the normal writing abilities of neurologically intact older adults.

The *Aphasia Diagnostic Profile* (ADP; Helm-Estabrooks, 1992), also described in Chapter 3, is one example of a test in which older adults participated in the standardization process. Data from 40 neurologically intact adults aged 20 to 99 years were included. Although 11 of these adults fell within the age range of 60 to 99, the test's author did not report the normative data by specific age groups. The following tasks make up the Writing subtest of the ADP: writing one's name; writing one's street address, city, state, zip code, birth date, Social Security number, and telephone number; signing one's name; and correctly dating the questionnaire. No additional tasks are included in the writing portion of this test. The ADP's test manual reports that neurologically intact adults in the standardization sample had a mean score of 24.4 (SD = 12.4) out of a possible 30 points. Thus, healthy adults ages 20 to 99 performed with an approximate average of 81% accuracy for the written items. A multidimensional scoring system is used for many subtests of the ADP, and the immediacy of a response is included as part of this scoring system. Although not reported in the test manual, it is possible that these individuals in the standardization sample accurately completed the writing tasks but were slow to respond, resulting in a lower score.

The *Arizona Battery for Communication Disorders of Dementia* (ABCD; Bayles & Tomoeda, 1993), also described in Chapter 3, is one of the few tests in which older adults were a separate control group. The mean age of these individuals was 70.44 years (SD = 17.07). Although handwriting is not formally included as part of this test, two subtests include drawing tasks: Generative Drawing and Figure Copying. For the Generative Drawing subtest, individuals draw a kite, a bucket, and a clock. For the Figure Copying subtest, individuals copy three abstract figures (e.g., circle with a cross through it). Both tasks are evaluated with a multidimensional scoring system to rate such aspects as shape, line approximations, and completeness. For the Generative Drawing subtest, older adults in the standardization sample received a mean score of 12.4 items correct (SD = 1.6) out of a total of 14 possible points, or 89% correct. For the Figure Copying subtest, the neurologically intact older adults achieved a mean of 11.4 (SD = 1.0) out of 12 possible points, or 95% correct. A second control group was made up of young adults, and on the Generative Drawing subtest, young adults did slightly better than older adults (mean score = 13.9; SD = 0.4; 99%). Average scores for older adults on the Figure Copying subtest did not differ significantly from those of the young adults (mean score = 11.8; SD = 0.8; 98%).

Research studies conducted on older adults' writing and drawing abilities indicate that age-related changes can occur in these areas. For example, the ability to copy simple geometrical figures such as circles and rectangles can decrease slightly with age; however, these drawings should in general be correct (Ericsson, Forssell, Holmèn, Viitanen, & Winblad, 1996). Greater reductions in accuracy occur when aging adults attempt to copy or draw more complex geometrical shapes. Specifically, older adults can have significant difficulty producing pentagons, rhombuses, or cubes (Ericsson et al., 1996). Older adults can generally write accurate spontaneous sentences, as found when participants wrote a sentence from the *Mini-Mental State Examination* (MMSE; Ericsson et al., 1996; Folstein, Folstein, & McHugh, 1975), yet there appears to be a decline in sentence complexity and the use of subordinating conjunctions (e.g., We are going out for dinner *after* we finish painting the living room; I enjoy reading *because* I feel I am learning new information; Bromley, 1991; Kemper, Greiner, Marquis, Prenovost, & Mitzner, 2001). Spelling accuracy can decline even for high-frequency words, particularly if they are difficult to spell (e.g., *restaurant, occasion*), and older adults may not always be aware that their spelling abilities have worsened (MacKay & Abrams, 1998). Aging adults reportedly rely more on the semantics of the sentence when writing homophones, whereas young adults generally choose the spelling consistent with the most regular spelling (Cortese, Balota, Sergent-Marshall, & Buckner, 2003). Some researchers report that because older adults have been exposed to more experiences during the course of their lives, their writing may contain increased vocabulary diversity, but other researchers report the opposite (Bromley, 1991). Declines in vocabulary diversity may occur because vocabulary acquired earlier in life and used more frequently is better retained than higher-level or less-frequently used vocabulary (Bromley, 1991).

In the study conducted by Burda (2007) described in previous chapters, adults aged 65 and older were divided into three separate age categories: Young-Old (M_{age} = 69.3 years), Middle-Old (M_{age} = 81.1 years), and Old-Old (M_{age} = 89.5 years). Ten participants were in the Young-Old and Old-Old groups and 11 were in the Middle-Old group. Participants completed a variety of writing tasks that can be clinically evaluated by SLPs, including writing the following biographical information: their name, their street address, city and state of residence, date of birth, and years of school completed. Other items included writing single words to dictation, writing the name of a pictured object, generating spontaneous sentences when provided a word, accurately filling out checks, and writing a grocery list. Results of this study, broken down by age groups, are included in **Table 6-1**.

Table 6-1

Task	Total*	Young-Old			Middle-Old			Old-Old		
		M	*SD*	%**	*M*	*SD*	%**	*M*	*SD*	%**
Biographical info	9	9.0	0.0	100	9.0	0.0	100	8.3	1.3	92
Words to dictation	10	9.9	0.3	99	9.8	0.4	98	9.9	0.3	99
Picture naming	10	10.0	0.0	100	9.9	0.3	99	9.9	0.3	99
Sentence generation	10	9.1	1.2	91	9.5	1.0	95	9.6	0.7	96
Completing checks	15	15.0	0.0	100	14.5	1.8	97	14.8	0.6	99
Writing grocery list	10	10.0	0.0	100	9.9	0.3	99	10.0	0.0	100

Mean Performance for Writing Tasks

Note: *refers to the total number of points possible. **refers to the percentage correct.
Source: Burda (2007).

As shown in Table 6-1, participants were able to complete all tasks with a high degree of accuracy. The lowest percentage of accuracy on any of these tasks was 91% on the sentence generation task in the Young-Old group. The majority of items were completed at a much higher degree of accuracy. No marked differences occurred across the age groups, and in some cases, those in the Old-Old group had higher mean scores than participants in the other two age groups. In addition, no statistically significant differences occurred in performance among the three age groups. It should be noted the sample size for this pilot study was small.

Older adults evidence motoric-related changes; however, application to real-life writing tasks is limited in the literature. Grip strength declines with age (Frederiksen, Hjelmborg, Mortensen, McGue, Vaupel, & Christensen, 2006), and movement can slow (Smith et al., 1999). Motor variability increases, possibly related to reduced initiation, control, force, and spatial coordination of movements (Contreras-Vidal, Teulings, & Stelmach, 1998). Variability is also evident in the duration of writing strokes, which are not as straight or as smooth as compared with younger adults' writing strokes (Contreras-Vidal et al., 1998).

The use of electronic communication among persons of all age groups has increased prolifically, and aging adults are no exception (Goodman, Syme, & Eisma, 2003). Older adults use the computer for many of the same reasons younger adults do: to use the Internet, e-mail family and friends, type various documents, conduct work-based activities, and play games (Champley, Scherz, Apel, & Burda, 2008; Echt, Morrell, & Park, 1998; Elias, Elias, Robin, & Gage, 1987; Goodman et al., 2003). Even if they are not familiar with computers initially, older adults are able to learn how to use computers and can retain this knowledge over time (Elias et al., 1987; Morrell, Park, Mayhorn, & Kelley, 2000; Morris, 1994). They are slower than younger adults when typing and editing documents (Czaja & Sharit, 1993; Elias et al., 1987) and can experience particular difficulty with moving the cursor, scrolling, tabbing, and using command characters that may be confusing (Elias et al., 1987; Mayhorn, Stronge, McLaughlin, & Rogers, 2004; Morris, 1994). Also, many technology products do not have features that can benefit older adults, such as easy-to-use menus and help sections or larger font sizes that allow them to adequately see what they are typing (Selwyn, Gorard, Furlong, & Madden, 2003).

In summary, based on information included in the normative data for adult language tests and in research studies, healthy older adults should be able to write personal information, including their name, address, date of birth, and Social Security number. In addition, older adults should be able to accurately write single words to dictation, write the name of a pictured item, accurately fill out checks, generate sentences spontaneously or when provided a word, and write a grocery list. They should be able to draw simple geometric shapes such as circles and rectangles but will likely have more difficulty with copying more complex figures, such as pentagons, rhombuses, or cubes. Aged adults may be slower motorically when writing and typing. They may also have difficulty spelling, and their writing complexity may be reduced. They should be able to use a computer, once they learn how, but they may experience difficulties if they are unable to see what they are typing, if applications are too complex, or with some of the movement-oriented tasks (e.g., scrolling, moving cursor). Although older adults' writing may change over time, there is nothing in the literature to suggest that their writing becomes markedly more difficult to produce or to read, or that significant declines occur in the accuracy of their written content. Thus, aging adults should be able to adequately communicate via writing. It is important to bear in mind that neurologically intact adults may be able to do far more than is reported here, and more research is needed to better document these abilities.

Factors Affecting Older Adults' Writing and Signs of Problems

Several factors can impact older adults' written abilities. Physical condition, educational level, and cognitive status have all been studied with respect to aging adults' writing. One study, conducted by Mitzner and Kemper (2003), investigated all of these issues. Females aged 78 to 91 participating in the Nun Study (Snowdon, Kemper, Mortimer, Greiner, Wekstein, & Markesbery, 1996) wrote autobiographical statements about their lives prior to entering the convent. Participants who were in better physical condition, had more education, and had higher cognitive functioning as measured by the MMSE (Folstein, Folstein, & McHugh, 1975) generated writing samples that had less-varied vocabulary, longer utterances, more clauses per utterance, more grammatically complex structures, and fewer fragments compared with participants who were in poorer physical condition, were not as highly educated, or had lower MMSE scores. Interestingly, age was not significantly correlated with any linguistic measures in this study. Mitzner and Kemper (2003) suggested that age-related writing changes may slow down or plateau later in life.

Other studies have also measured the effects of education and cognition on writing skills. Older adults' abilities to copy circles and rectangles, write their names, and write sentences from dictation do not tend to vary based on the number of years spent in school (Ericsson et al., 1996). More complex tasks, such as copying pentagons and cubes and writing a spontaneous sentence, do appear to be related to the level of education (Ericsson et al., 1996). That is, those with more education likely have better performance on these specific tasks compared with individuals who have less education.

Studies in cognition and writing have focused on working memory and attention. Writing requires a significant amount of working memory (Hoskyn & Swanson, 2003; Olive, 2004). Older adults, however, have declines in working memory that lead to less storage and processing capacity (Hoskyn & Swanson, 2003). Thus, more resources are needed for older adults to generate ideas and turn these ideas into written output. The end result is writing that is structurally less complex (Hoskyn & Swanson, 2003). For example, written narratives may have events that are not thoroughly temporally or causally related (Hoskyn & Swanson, 2003). Decline in attention can lead to spelling errors (Neils, Roeltgen, & Greer, 1995). This is notable because language impairments are typically thought to be the primary cause of spelling difficulties.

Adequate vision is crucial to see what one is writing or typing (Hawthorn, 2000; Ryan, Anas, Beamer, & Bajorek, 2003). Several age-related changes in vision can occur, including declines in visual acuity and contrast sensitivity (i.e., detecting differences in illumination levels) and the development of presbyopia, the gradual loss of the eyes' ability to focus actively on nearby objects (Glasser & Campbell, 1998). Glare can also be an issue (Hagerstrom-Portnoy, Schneck, & Brabyn, 1999), and it can be particularly problematic when older adults are using computers. Reduced vision can have clinical implications. For example, impaired vision can lead to lower scores on the MMSE (Jagger, Clarke, Anderson, & Battcock, 1992), which is frequently used as a screening tool in medical settings, and healthcare professionals could incorrectly conclude that older patients have impaired cognitive abilities.

Because of these vision changes, most older adults need to wear corrective lenses (Desai, Pratt, Lentzner, & Robinson, 2001). If they do not have glasses or contact lenses, or the prescription for these items is no longer sufficient, individuals generally have well-developed underlying motor programs that can compensate to some degree for reduced vision (Graham & Weintraub, 1996; Stelmach & Teulings, 1983). Regardless, vision changes need to be properly addressed so that older adults' writing and legibility are not negatively impacted.

Familiarity with specific tasks and the presence of external visual stimuli may affect aging adults' writing. Older adults need more time to plan and execute their movements when writing tasks are unfamiliar or difficult (Dixon, Kurzman, & Friesen, 1993; Portier, van Galen, & Meulenbroek, 1990; Rogers, Meyer, Walker, & Fisk, 1998). For example, older adults in the early stages of learning how to use a computer would need more time to type and send e-mail. In contrast, writing a grocery list would be a familiar and relatively easy activity to complete. Preliminary data suggest that the presence of external visual stimuli may have an adverse effect on older adults' writing. In a study measuring younger and older adults' movements when writing a string of letters, the inclusion of lines on the writing surface (similar to lined paper) reduced the efficiency of older adults' movements (Slavin, Phillips, & Bradshaw, 1996). Although only the movements were measured and accuracy of the content was not, it is possible that the presence of the lines led to a reduction in the older adults' attentional abilities. More research needs to be done to better determine the effects of external visual stimuli on older adults' writing.

There are signs that can indicate aging adults are having trouble writing. The term *dysgraphia* is generally used to refer to difficulties with writing, spelling, and/or typing (N. Graham, 2000; Neils-Strunjas, Groves-Wright, Mashima, & Harnish, 2006). Obviously, older adults who have overt complaints of not being able to write or type, that their writing has significantly changed, or that they are experiencing pain when writing or typing, such as in the case of arthritis (Kauranen, Vuotikka, & Hakala, 2005; Zhang, Niu, Kelly-Hayes, Chaisson, Aliabadi, & Felson, 2002), should see their physician. When older adults demonstrate difficulty writing, spelling, typing, and/or drawing that differs from their typical performance, it is frequently a sign of an underlying neuropathology (Longstaff & Heath, 1997). Writing problems can suggest cognitive-linguistic disruptions, such as in the case of Alzheimer's disease (Harnish & Neils-Strunjas, 2008; Neils et al., 1995), or the presence of motor disorders, such as amyotrophic lateral sclerosis (Weber, Eisen, Stewart, & Hirota, 2000), multiple sclerosis, or Parkinson's disease (Longstaff & Heath, 2003).

Persons with Parkinson's disease or dementia can be particularly susceptible to dysgraphia. The presence of micrographia, or abnormally small handwriting, is common with Parkinson's disease (Ondo & Satija, 2007; Yorkston, Miller, & Strand, 2004). Damage to the basal ganglia causes the muscles to become rigid, and individuals' overall range of movement is reduced (Olivera, Gurd, Nixon, Marshall, & Passingham, 1997). Micrographia can lead to such diminished legibility that the reader may not be able to determine what was written.

Individuals with dementia can exhibit a variety of writing, spelling, and/or drawing difficulties. For example, an inability to copy specific geometric shapes, specifically if the shape is something other than a circle, is considered an early sign of dementia (Ericsson et al., 1996). Copying pentagons and cubes in particular seems to be the most sensitive to cognitive decline, while copying circles and writing one's name appears to be the least sensitive (Ericsson et al., 1996). Writing abilities can vary significantly in dementia. Many people in the mild stages (i.e., early stages) have difficulty writing complete spontaneous sentences (Ericsson et al., 1996). In contrast, some individuals in the mild stages may be able to write a paragraph; however, spelling errors are usually present (Domenico, 1990). Certain items are reportedly difficult for persons with mild-to-moderate dementia, including lengthier words, low-frequency words, homophones, and nonwords (Harnish & Neils-Strunjas, 2008; Neils-Strunjas et al., 2006). Not surprisingly, performance on written tasks tends to worsen as dementia becomes more severe (Groves-Wright, Neils-Strunjas, Burnett, & O'Neill, 2004). Groves-Wright and colleagues (2004) found that semantic paragraphias on written confrontation naming tasks increased with advancing dementia. They also reported that persons with moderate dementia performed more poorly on written fluency tasks (e.g., writing the name of as many animals as possible in one minute) than those with mild dementia. The abilities to write sentences to dictation and sign one's name appear to be retained longer than other writing abilities in individuals with dementia (Ericsson et al., 1996). At the narrative level (e.g., picture description), persons with Alzheimer's disease tend to have difficulty fully describing the picture and exhibit semantic paragraphias (e.g., "lengthy station" written to indicate a pier; Groves-Wright et al., 2004; Horner, Heyman, Dawson, & Rogers, 1988). Written narratives also tend to be shorter, include repetitive content and restricted vocabulary, and have irrelevant information and content word errors (Harnish & Neils-Strunjas, 2008).

Additional signs of writing problems that warrant an appointment with a physician include shakiness, tremors, and/or weakness when writing, or difficulty gripping writing utensils. Seeing a doctor can be warranted if others notice that older adults' written output is nonsensical, the content does not match the task, or if more sentence fragments are written than complete sentences (Small, Lyons, & Kemper, 1997). Aging adults who are unable to finish written activities or who ask others to complete writing tasks they previously were able to perform (e.g., filling out checks) should also be seen by a medical professional. In some cases, the older persons may need to be seen by an optometrist to have their vision assessed; however, if improvements in writing are not seen after that, then feedback from other medical professionals should be sought. If any of the writing difficulties discussed here are reported or observed, older adults should be referred to their physician, with possible additional referrals to other specialists such as neurologists, SLPs, or occupational therapists.

Strategies to Help Older Adults' Writing

Strategies exist that can aid older adults in their written expression. Because fine motor abilities and working memory can decline with age, providing older adults with as much time as they need can aid their writing (Bromley, 1991; Jones & Bayen, 1998) and computer-based activities

(Elias et al., 1987). The lack of time constraints lets aged adults determine exactly what it is they would like to write or type, and then allows them to focus on their motoric output. Practice can also improve written performance (Dixon et al., 1993; Portier et al., 1990) and proficiency on the computer (Elias et al., 1987; Gist, Rosen, & Schwoerer, 1988), and it can be particularly beneficial with unfamiliar tasks (Portier et al., 1990). Managing any vision changes may help older adults who have challenges seeing what they are writing or typing. If they are having difficulties gripping a writing utensil, older adults may do better if they use pens or pencils with a wider diameter (e.g., wider pen instead of a slim pen) or if a rubber gripper is placed around the writing utensil. Older adults in the initial stages of learning how to use a computer should be provided with clear and extensive explanations of the equipment as well as the differences between traditional typing and word processing on a computer; written materials and audio-recorded materials should be provided as adjuncts (Elias et al., 1987). Older adults also find it helpful to watch a model demonstrate a task before they complete a computer activity themselves (Gist et al., 1988). Aging adults can employ other helpful strategies when using the computer, such as making use of spelling and grammar checks (MacKay & Abrams, 1998). As far as the content of writing, older adults may benefit from memory strategies if they are having difficulty remembering what they want to write. For example, those who cannot remember what they want to buy at the grocery store should make a list throughout the week.

Quick Facts

- General Writing Abilities of Neurologically Intact Older Adults:
    - Write personal information, such as name, address, date of birth, and Social Security number
    - Write single words to dictation
    - Write the name of a pictured item
    - Fill out checks
    - Generate written sentences spontaneously or when provided with a word
    - Write a grocery list
    - Copy simple geometric shapes such as circles and rectangles
    - Demonstrate difficulty with copying more complex geometric figures, such as pentagons, rhombuses, or cubes
    - May write more slowly
    - May have difficulty spelling and a reduction in the complexity of their writing

- Can use a computer once they learn how but may experience difficulties with movement-oriented tasks, such as scrolling or moving the cursor
- Can have difficulty using a computer if they have vision problems that prevent them from seeing what they are typing or if the applications are too complex
- In general, should be able to communicate adequately when writing

- Factors That Can Negatively Affect Older Adults' Writing:
  - Poor physical condition
  - Lower levels of education
  - Lower cognitive functioning
  - Presence of age-related vision changes, such as visual acuity declines, reduced contrast sensitivity, and presbyopia
  - Unfamiliar writing task
  - Presence of external visual stimuli (e.g., lines on paper)
- Signs That an Older Adult Should Be Referred to a Speech-Language Pathologist or Other Medical Professionals:
  - Overt complaints of not being able to write or type, that writing has significantly changed, or pain occurs when writing or typing
  - Difficulty copying geometric shapes, particularly cubes and pentagons. Circles are easiest to copy, even for persons with dementia
  - Difficulty typing on a computer
  - Difficulty writing spontaneous sentences or paragraphs
  - Problems writing lengthier words, low-frequency words, and nonwords
  - Presence of tremors, shakiness, weakness, or micrographia when writing
  - Difficulty holding a writing utensil
  - Content does not match the task or the written output is nonsensical
  - Inability to finish written activities or assign others writing tasks they were previously able to complete (e.g., filling out checks)

(Note: If compromised vision is suspected, refer the individual to an optometrist.)

- Strategies That Can Help Older Adults' Writing:
  - Allow as much time as needed to write or type
  - Encourage older adults to practice writing or typing
  - Provide older adults in the initial stages of learning how to use a computer with clear and extensive explanations of the equipment and the differences between traditional typing and word processing on a computer; written

materials and audio-recorded materials should be provided as adjuncts
- Encourage older adults to make use of functions such as spelling and grammar checks on the computer
- Manage any vision changes
- Provide a writing utensil with a wider diameter or a rubber gripper around the writing utensil that makes it easier to grip
- Encourage older adults to implement memory strategies if they are unable to recall what they want to write, such as making a grocery list throughout the week versus trying to generate a list all at one time

Discussion Questions

1. What are the reasons that spelling abilities can decline in older age?
2. How does performance on the clock-drawing test differ between normal aging adults and adults with neurological disorders (e.g., dementia)?
3. Take time to search Web sites that older adults might use in order to gain health-oriented information, including the American Speech-Language-Hearing Association's Web site. Based on your research, which Web sites do you believe would be more difficult for older adults to navigate? Which ones would they be able to navigate more easily? What issues factored into your decisions?
4. What are the legal implications if older adults cannot sign their names to important legal or financial documents? How can this issue be addressed?

References

Alamargot, D., & Chanquoy, L. (2001). Through the models of writing. Dordrecht, Netherlands: Kluwer Academic Publishers.

Andersen, D. W. (1969). What makes writing legible? Elementary School Journal, 69, 364–369.

Bayles, K. A., & Tomoeda, C. K. (1993). Arizona Battery for Communication Disorders of Dementia. Tucson, AZ: Canyonlands Publishing.

Blanton, D. J., & Degenais, P. A. (2007). Comparison of language skills of adjudicated and nonadjudicated adolescent males and females. Language, Speech, and Hearing Services in Schools, 38, 309–314.

Bromley, D. B. (1991). Aspects of written language production over adult life. Psychology and Aging, 6, 296–308.

Burda, A. N. (2007). Communication changes in healthy aging adults. Adele Whitenack Davis Research in Gerontology Award, University of Northern Iowa, Cedar Falls, IA.

Champley, J., Scherz, J. W., Apel, K., & Burda, A. (2008). A preliminary analysis of reading materials and strategies used by older adults. *Communication Disorders Quarterly, 29,* 131–140.

Contreras-Vidal, J. L., Teulings, H. L., & Stelmach, G. E. (1998). Elderly subjects are impaired in spatial coordination in fine motor control. *Acta Psychologica, 100,* 25–35.

Cortese, M. J., Balota, D. A., Sergent-Marshall, S. D., & Buckner, R. L. (2003). Sublexical, lexical, and semantic influences in spelling: Exploring the effects of age, Alzheimer's disease and primary semantic impairment. *Neuropsychologia, 41,* 952–967.

Czaja, S., & Sharit, J. (1993). Age differences in the performance of computer-based work. *Psychology and Aging, 8,* 59–67.

Desai, M., Pratt, L. A., Lentzner, H., & Robinson, K. N. (2001). Trends in vision and hearing among older Americans. *Aging Trends, No.2.* Hyattsville, MD: National Center for Health Statistics.

Dixon, R. A., Kurzman, D., & Friesen, I. C. (1993). Handwriting performance in younger and older adults: Age, familiarity, and practice effects. *Psychology and Aging, 8,* 360–370.

Domenico, R. A. (1990). Verbal communication impairment in dementia research frontiers in language and cognition. In T. Zandi & R. J. Ham (Eds.), *New directions in understanding dementia and Alzheimer's disease* (pp. 79–88). New York: Plenum Press.

Echt, K. V., Morrell, R. W., & Park, D. C. (1998). Effects of age and training format on basic computer skill acquisition in older adults. *Educational Gerontology, 24,* 3–25.

Elias, P. K., Elias, M. F., Robin, M. A., & Gage, P. (1987). Acquisition of word-processing skills by younger, middle-age, and older adults. *Psychology and Aging, 2,* 340–348.

Ericsson, K., Forssell, L. G., Holmèn, K., Viitanen, M., & Winblad, B. (1996). Copying and handwriting ability in the screening of cognitive dysfunction in old age. *Archives of Gerontology and Geriatrics, 22,* 103–121.

Folstein, M. F., Folstein, S. E., & McHugh, P. R. (1975). Mini-mental state: A practical method for grading the cognitive state of patients for the clinician. *Journal of Psychiatric Research, 12,* 189–198.

Frederiksen, H., Hjelmborg, J., Mortensen, J., McGue, M., Vaupel, J. W., & Christensen, K. (2006). Age trajectories of grip strength: Cross-sectional and longitudinal data among 8, 342 Danes aged 46–102. *Annals of Epidemiology, 16,* 554–562.

Glasser, A., & Campbell, M. C. W. (1998). Presbyopia and the optical changes in the human crystalline lens with age. *Vision Research, 38,* 209–229.

Gist, M., Rosen, B., & Schwoerer, C. (1988). The influence of training method and trainee age on the acquisition of computer skills. *Personnel Psychology, 41,* 255–265.

Goodman, J., Syme, A., & Eisma, R. (2003). Older adults' use of computers: A survey. *Proceedings of Human-Computer Interaction Conference: Designing for Society, 2,* 25–28.

Graham, N. (2000). Dysgraphia in dementia. *Neurocase, 6,* 365–376.

Graham, S., & Weintraub, N. (1996). A review of handwriting research: Progress and prospects from 1980 to 1994. *Educational Psychology Review, 8,* 7–87.

Groves-Wright, K., Neils-Strunjas, J., Burnett, R., & O'Neill, M. J. (2004). A comparison of verbal and written language in Alzheimer's disease. *Journal of Communication Disorders, 37,* 109–130.

Hagerstrom-Portnoy, G., Schneck, M. E., & Brabyn, J. A. (1999). Seeing into old age: Vision function beyond acuity. *Optometry and Vision Science, 76,* 141–158.

Harnish, S. M., & Neils-Strunjas, J. (2008). In search of meaning: Reading and writing in Alzheimer's disease. *Seminars in Speech and Language, 29,* 44–59.

Hawthorn, D. (2000). Possible implications of aging for interface designers. *Interacting With Computers, 12,* 507–528.

Helm-Estabrooks, N. (1992). *Aphasia Diagnostic Profile*. Dedham, MA: AliMed.

Helm-Estabrooks, N. (2001). *Cognitive Linguistic Quick Test*. San Antonio, TX: The Psychological Corporation.

Horner, J., Heyman, A., Dawson, D., & Rogers, H. (1988). The relationship of agraphia to the severity of dementia in Alzheimer's disease. *Archives in Neurology, 45*, 760–763.

Hoskyn, M., & Swanson, L. H. (2003). The relationship between working memory and writing in younger and older adults. *Reading and Handwriting: An Interdisciplinary Journal, 16*, 759–784.

Huber, R. A., & Headrick, A. M. (1999). *Handwriting identification: Facts and fundamentals*. Boca Raton, FL: CRC Press.

Jagger, C., Clarke, M., Anderson, J., & Battcock, T. (1992). Misclassifications of dementia by the Mini-Mental State Examination: Are education and social class the only factors? *Age and Ageing, 21*, 404–411.

Jones, B. D., & Bayen, U. J. (1998). Teaching older adults to use computers: Recommendations based on cognitive aging research. *Educational Gerontology, 24*, 675–689.

Kauranen, K., Vuotikka, P., & Hakala, M. (2005). Motor performance of the hand in patients with rheumatoid arthritis. *Annals of Rheumatology Disorders, 59*, 812–826.

Keenan, J. S., & Brassell, E.G. (1975). *Aphasia Language Performance Scales*. Murfreesboro, TN: Pinnacle Press.

Kemper, S., Greiner, L. H., Marquis, J. G., Prenovost, K., & Mitzner, T. L. (2001). Language decline across the life span: Findings from the Nun Study. *Psychology and Aging, 16*, 227–239.

Kertesz, A. (2006). *Western Aphasia Battery–Revised*. San Antonio, TX: Harcourt Assessment, Inc.

Kopeenhaver, K. (2007). *Forensic document examination: Principles and practices*. Totowa, NJ: Humana Press.

Longstaff, M. G., & Heath, R. A. (1997). Space-time invariance in adult handwriting. *Acta Psychologica, 97*, 210–214.

Longstaff, M. G., & Heath, R. A. (2003). The influence of motor system degradation on the control of handwriting movements: A dynamical systems analysis. *Human Movement Science, 22*, 91–110.

MacKay, D. G., & Abrams, L. (1998). Age-linked declines in retrieving orthographic knowledge: Empirical, practical, and theoretical implications. *Psychology and Aging, 13*, 647–662.

Mayhorn, C. B., Stronge, A. J., McLaughlin, A., & Rogers, W. A. (2004). Older adults, computer training, and the systems approach: A formula for success. *Educational Gerontology, 30*, 185–203.

Mitzner, T. L., & Kemper, S. (2003). Oral and written language in late adulthood: Findings from the Nun Study. *Experimental Aging Research, 29*, 457–474.

Morrell, R. W., Park, D. C., Mayhorn, C. B., & Kelley, C. L. (2000). Effects of age and instructions on teaching older adults to use ELDERCOMM, an electronic bulletin board system. *Educational Gerontology, 26*, 221–235.

Morris, M. J. (1994). Computer training needs of older adults. *Educational Gerontology, 20*, 541–556.

Neils, J., Roeltgen, D. P., & Greer, A. (1995). Spelling and attention in early Alzheimer's disease: Evidence for impairment of the graphemic buffer. *Brain and Language, 49*, 27–49.

Neils-Strunjas, J., Groves-Wright, K., Mashima, P., & Harnish, S. (2006). Dysgraphia in Alzheimer's disease: A review for clinical and research purposes. *Journal of Speech, Language, and Hearing Research, 49*, 1313–1330.

Olive, T. (2004). Working memory in writing: Empirical evidence from the dual-task technique. *European Psychologist, 9*, 32–42.

Olivera, R. M., Gurd, J. M., Nixon, P., Marshall, J. C., & Passingham, R. E. (1997). Micrographia in Parkinson's disease: The effect of providing external cues. *Journal of Neurology, Neurosurgery, and Psychiatry, 63*, 429–433.

Ondo, W. G., & Satija, P. (2007). Withdrawal of visual feedback improves micrographia in Parkinson's disease. *Movement Disorders, 22*, 2130–2131.

Portier, S. J., van Galen, G. P., & Meulenbroek, R. G. (1990). Practice and the dynamics of handwriting performance: Evidence for a shift of motor programming load. *Journal of Motor Behavior, 22*, 474–492.

Rogers, W., Meyer, B., Walker, N., & Fisk, A. (1998). Functional limitations to daily living tasks in the aged: A focus group. *Human Factors, 40*, 111–125.

Rubin, N., & Henderson, S. E. (1982). Two sides of the same coin? Variations in teaching methods and failure to learn to write. *Special Education: Forward Trends, 9*, 17–24.

Ryan, E. B., Anas, A. P., Beamer, M., & Bajorek, S. (2003). Coping with age-related vision loss in everyday reading activities. *Educational Gerontology, 29*, 37–54.

Schuell, H. (1973). *Minnesota Test for the Differential Diagnosis of Aphasia* (2nd ed., revised by J. W. Sefer). Minneapolis: University of Minnesota Press.

Selwyn, N., Gorard, S., Furlong, J., & Madden, L. (2003). Older adults' use of information and communications technology in everyday life. *Ageing and Society, 23*, 561–582.

Slavin, M. J., Phillips, J. G., & Bradshaw, J. L. (1996). Visual cues and the handwriting of older adults: A kinematic analysis. *Psychology and Aging, 3*, 521–526.

Small, J. A., Lyons, K. A., & Kemper, S. (1997). Grammatical abilities in Parkinson's disease: Evidence from written sentences. *Neuropsychologia, 35*, 1571–1576.

Smith, C. D., Umberger, G. H., Manning, E. L., Slevin, J. T., Wekstein, D. R., Schmitt, F. A., et al. (1999). Critical decline in fine motor hand movements in human aging. *Neurology, 53*, 1458–1461.

Snowdon, D. A., Kemper, S. J., Mortimer, J. A., Greiner, L. H., Wekstein, D. R., & Markesbery, W. R. (1996). Linguistic ability in early life and cognitive function and Alzheimer's disease in later life: Findings from the Nun Study. *Journal of the American Medical Association, 275*, 528–532.

Stelmach, G., & Teulings, H. (1983). Response characteristics of prepared and restructured handwriting. *Acta Psychologica, 54*, 51–67.

Tomchek, S. D., & Schneck, C. M. (2005). Evaluation of handwriting. In A. Henderson & C. Pehoski (Eds.), *Hand function in the child: Foundations for remediation* (pp. 293–320). St. Louis, MO: Elsevier Health Sciences.

Tynjälä, P., Mason, L., & Lonka, K. (2001). *Writing as a learning tool: Integrating theory and practice*. Dordrecht, Netherlands: Kluwer Academic Publishers.

Walton, J. (1997). Handwriting changes due to aging and Parkinson's syndrome. *Forensic Science International, 88*, 197–214.

Weber, M., Eisen, A., Stewart, H., & Hirota, N. (2000). The split hand in ALS has a cortical basis. *Journal of the Neurological Sciences, 180*, 66–70.

Wellingham-Jones, P. (1989). *The mind/body connection: Neurophysiological basis for handwriting* (2nd ed.). Tehama, CA: PJW Publishing.

Wright, E. (1990). Evaluating the special role of time in the control of handwriting. *Acta Psychologica, 82*, 5–52.

Yorkston, K. M., Miller, R. M., & Strand, E. A. (2004). *Management of speech and swallowing disorders in degenerative diseases* (2nd ed.). Austin, TX: Pro-Ed.

Zhang, Y., Niu, J., Kelly-Hayes, M., Chaisson, C. E., Aliabadi, P., & Felson, D. T. (2002). Prevalence of symptomatic hand osteoarthritis and its impact on functional status among the elderly. *American Journal of Epidemiology, 156*, 1021–1027.

Chapter 7

Voice and Motor Speech Abilities

Todd A. Bohnenkamp, PhD, CCC-SLP

Carlin F. Hageman, PhD, CCC-SLP

Introduction

Our voices undergo significant change as we age. Although much research has been done on changes in the larynx in aging adults, the exact mechanisms responsible for the changes in the elderly voice are not well known. Many aspects of phonation are influenced in aging, and they are evaluated using perceptual ratings, videostroboscopic ratings, acoustic measures, and physiologic measures. Studies have focused on the histology, neurology, and myology of phonation, and gender differences between aging speakers have also been examined. Although a great deal of the literature focuses on voice, research has also been conducted on motor speech abilities in the aged. Some of the changes in speech processes are related not only to age, but also to behaviors across the life span, particularly smoking.

This chapter discusses voice and motor speech abilities in older adults, factors that can negatively affect these abilities, signs that warrant referral to a speech-language pathologist (SLP) or other medical professionals, and strategies that can help aging adults' voice and motor speech abilities. An additional section discusses the various tools available that can be used for assessment and treatment purposes. A list of "Quick Facts" summarizes key points from this chapter.

Older Adults' General Voice and Motor Speech Abilities

Several investigators have reported voice changes with age (Baken, 2005; Brown, Morris, & Michel, 1989; McGlone & Hollien, 1963; Ramig & Ringel, 1983). These changes include diminished volume, breathiness, relatively high pitch, diminished flexibility, and tremulousness. Fundamental frequency (F_0) decreases with maturity and then increases in older age. In addition, older speakers have a decreased phonation range. Increased jitter and shimmer values have been reported by some researchers. These changes may be related to physiological differences in speakers versus chronological differences, but in general, they indicate that phonatory stability decreases with age. Baken (2005) argues that older speakers' phonation is less stable and less well controlled than that of younger speakers.

The vocal tract itself does not change its overall size due to the aging process, but it appears that the oral cavity may enlarge somewhat while the pharyngeal cavity does not. This may lower the first formant (F1) a bit in older speakers. The literature suggests that the variability of vocal production (shimmer and jitter) may increase with age and that pitch in older males may rise. Breathiness becomes more concentrated in the higher spectrum in older women because the glottal gap shifts from a posterior one to an anterior one. Velopharyngeal function and articulation (except for the lower F1) do not appear to change with age. References to changes in motor speech abilities or voice that can be attributed to age alone (e.g., presbylarynges, the age-related changes in the structure of the larynx or presbyphonia, the perceptual characteristics of presbylarynges) are not common in the literature (Woo, Casper, Colton, & Brewer, 1992). A diagnosis of presbylarynges should be made only following careful exclusion of other etiologies.

Factors Affecting Voice and Motor Speech Abilities and Signs of Problems

Acoustic signs (cues) of the aging voice are a product of the physiology of the system. These changes are in the respiratory, laryngeal, articulatory, and resonatory systems and are the result of histological and behavioral changes (Sataloff, 1998). There is no model that adequately captures changes in the acoustic properties of voice and their physical etiologies that would make it possible to differentiate between pathological voices and normal aging voices. There are, however, signs that can indicate potential phonatory problems in the aged.

Respiratory Factors

The respiratory system is influenced by changes in the musculoskeletal system that make the system stiffer and the muscles weaker. The lung tissue itself undergoes changes that result in air trapping. The end result of these changes is that older individuals tend to be more inefficient breathers. This is especially noticeable in their tidal breathing, which takes place at higher lung volumes; however, this usually does not come into play for speech unless a person is compromised by disease, which makes compensation for age-associated changes difficult.

Several factors can affect older adults' respiratory function. In general, identifying changes in the respiratory abilities of individuals as they age is complicated. The respiratory challenges can be caused by aging itself, by a disease state, such as respiratory illness (e.g., tuberculosis, emphysema, congestive heart failure), or by injuries to the respiratory system as a result of smoking or exposure to industrial and environmental toxins. These conditions negatively influence respiration; however, even in healthy adults, pulmonary function decreases with age (Ayres, 1990; Chan & Welsh, 1998; Janssens, Pache, & Nicod, 1999). Respiratory system changes are more pronounced in older women than in males (Burrows, Cline, Knudson, Taussig, & Lebowitz, 1983; Hoit & Hixon, 1987; Hoit, Hixon, Altman, & Morgan, 1989).

The primary respiratory system changes associated with increased age include decreased elastic recoil, decreased compliance of the chest wall (i.e., rib cage, diaphragm, and abdomen), and reduced strength of the respiratory muscles. The loss of recoil is related to the calcification of the costal and rib/vertebral articulations and narrowing of the intervertebral spaces (Crapo, 1993; Murray, 1986). In addition to the calcification, osteoporosis of the vertebrae can result in a wedging or crushing of vertebral fractures, which leads to dorsal kyphosis ("hunchback") and increased anterior–posterior dimension of the chest wall ("barrel chest"). Kahane (1980) also observed that the bony thorax stiffens with age.

Adequate compliance and elasticity of the pulmonary system are essential for efficient speech breathing. Pierce and Ebert (1965) reported that the pleural membranes lose elasticity with increased age. Speakers maintain the tongue pressure necessary for speech by integrating passive forces in the respiratory system (e.g., recoil forces) with muscular effort via the respiratory musculature (Hixon, Goldman, & Mead, 1973; Hixon, Mead, & Goldman, 1976). Increased lung volumes result in increased passive forces available for speech production.

Low lung volumes lead to decreased passive forces, subsequently requiring muscular effort to maintain adequate subglottal pressures.

Reduced elasticity (recoil) in the system can also result in decreased passive forces, requiring more effort on the part of the speaker. Due to the reduced elasticity in the pleural membranes as well as the stiffening of the thorax, older speakers need higher lung volumes to create more passive force to drive the speaking mechanism. Many older speakers have muscular weakness, however. Dhar, Shastri, and Lenora (1976) and McKeown (1965) reported that speaking at higher lung volumes may be compromised in older speakers due to muscular weakness. Older speakers may compensate by recruiting more muscle activity for inspiration and expiration, but the actual weakness of a muscle or a reduced number of muscle fibers may prevent successful compensation. For example, diaphragmatic strength decreases with age (Polkey, Harris, Hughes, Hamengard, Lyons, & Moxham, 1997). Tolep, Higgins, Muza, Criner, and Kelsen (1995) reported reduced diaphragmatic strength in elderly men who were classified as fit.

In addition, there is a loss in the cross-sectional area of the intercostal muscles indicating muscle atrophy and probable weakness (Brown & Hasser, 1996; Tolep & Kelsen, 1993). When muscle atrophy occurs, the respiratory system becomes less elastic and can result in a reduction of vital capacity (Brown et al., 1989; Hoit & Hixon, 1987; Kahane, 1980, 1981, 1983, 1987, 1988, 1990; Kendall, 2007; Sperry & Klich, 1992). As a result of the increased muscular effort for successful compensation, older adults may have less physical reserve to deal with illness when it occurs. Air trapping, muscular weakness, and loss of structural flexibility lead to residual volume increases by 50% between ages 20 and 70, at the same time that vital capacity decreases to 75% of an individual's peak values. Subsequently, the elderly breathe using higher lung volumes because their functional residual capacity is increased compared with younger adults (i.e., increased resting expiratory level) and results in decreased passive forces available for speech. A result is that 60-year-old males can expend 20% more energy during tidal breathing than do 20-year-olds (Janssens et al., 1999).

Respiratory muscle strength may also be related to the nutritional status or weight of an individual. There are negative correlations between maximal inspiratory and expiratory pressures with body mass and weight (Enright, Kronmal, Manolio, Schenker, & Hyatt, 1994). In addition, undernourished patients display decreased maximal voluntary ventilation and reduced respiratory muscle strength (Arora & Rochester, 1982).

Changes in the strength of the muscles of the respiratory system dovetail well with existing literature showing that peripheral musculature strength declines with age (i.e., > age 65; Bassey & Harries, 1993; Lexell, 1997). Interestingly, maximal inspiratory and expiratory pressures are strongly correlated to hand-grip strength (Enright et al., 1994). Explanations for the decrease in muscular force include, but are not limited to: decreased muscle mass (both cross-sectional muscle fiber area and the number of muscle fibers), reduced type II or "fast twitch fibers," altered neuromuscular junction, and denervated muscle fibers, specifically type II.

The peripheral airways of the respiratory system must remain patent for optimal gas exchange. A significant portion of these airways do not contribute to gas exchange in older speakers due to a loss of airway-supporting tissue (Janssens, Pache, & Nicod, 1999). A consequence of the reduction in supporting tissues around the airways is a tendency for the small airways (<2 mm) to collapse, narrowing the lumina and resulting in decreased flow rates during expiration. The terminal bronchioles (pathways) narrow upon expiration, whereas the terminal air spaces remain inflated, resulting in air trapping (Meyer, 2005). Premature closure of the airways may, therefore, occur during tidal breathing (Crapo, 1993). In addition, the elderly have fewer alveoli and fewer capillaries per alveolus. As a result, older individuals experience decreased ventilation/perfusion within the alveoli, leading to lower oxygen pressures throughout the arterial system. Again, elderly persons who compensate for these respiratory challenges may find that compensation is unattainable when diseases or injuries create additional demands upon respiration or attention. For example, persons with severe chronic obstructive pulmonary disease (COPD) may demonstrate breathlessness, shorter utterance lengths, and poor ability to control speaking loudness. As a whole, these changes have been designated as "senile emphysema" (Verbeken, Cauberghs, & Mertens, 1992).

Not only do older speakers have difficulty with compensating for muscular and structural changes, they must also deal with decreased sensitivity to hypercapnia (too much carbon dioxide in the blood) or hypoxia (too little oxygen in the blood). Either of these conditions might result in an inability to adequately monitor blood values during heart failure or airway obstruction (e.g., COPD; Janssens et al., 1999). Overall, gas exchange is preserved at both rest and activity in spite of these differences. If, however, older speakers develop an infection or heart failure, these changes can result in decompensation of a task (e.g., speaking).

Additionally, asthma in the elderly is an often underdiagnosed condition. This is interesting considering that hospitalizations for asthma are highest in individuals older than 65 and its presence provides another potential source for decompensation of supposedly intact abilities (e.g., swallowing). During the 1980s an increase in asthma death rates for individuals over the age of 65 was reported, especially for those with co-occurring diseases (Evans, Mullally, Wilson, Gergen, Rosenberg, Grauman et al., 1987; Moorman & Mannino 2001; Robin, 1988; Sly, 1984).

Laryngeal Factors

The larynx has been documented to change with age. These changes include ossification of the laryngeal cartilages, muscular decline, and postmenopausal changes (Boulet & Oddens, 1996; Hirano, Kurita, & Nakashima, 1983; R. Ryan, McDonald, & Devine, 1956). Ossification and tissue degeneration in the larynx are more pronounced in older males than in females (Kahane, 1987, 1988, 1990).

Listeners can distinguish between young and older voices based on speech and other productions (Gorham-Rowan & Laures-Gore, 2006; Linville & Fisher, 1985a; Linville & Korabic, 1986; Ptacek & Sander, 1966; Ptacek, Sander, Maloney, & Jackson, 1966; W. Ryan & Burk, 1974; Shipp & Hollien, 1969). These distinguishing cues are not only acoustic in nature but can include phrasing, voice breaks, vitality, hesitancy, vocal tremor, imprecise consonants, and reduced rate or articulation (W. Ryan & Burk, 1974). Additional characteristics include hoarseness, voice breaks, and lowering of pitch (Benjamin, 1981; Ptacek & Sander, 1966; Ptacek et al., 1966; W. Ryan & Burk, 1974). For example, F_0 decreases with age until the fifth decade of life and subsequently rises gradually (Sataloff, Rosen, Hawkshaw, & Spiegel, 1997).

Orlikoff (1990) reported significant differences in acoustic variables between young, older, and atherosclerotic speakers but did not include F_0 differences. Jitter and shimmer values were significantly higher in older and atherosclerotic speakers, which may be indicative of a time of "elderly individualism" after the sixth decade of life, similar to the changes seen during prepubescence. Orlikoff and others (Brown et al., 1989; Linville & Fisher, 1985a) stated that increased vocal variability on acoustic measures might be a better approach to understanding changes in voice with age versus the use of group means. Specifically, hoarseness is a poor cue for senescent voice and that variability (in F_0 standard deviation) and elevated jitter and shimmer values are apparent both in pathological cases and in the voices of typically aging adults (Davis, 1979; Iwata, 1972; Iwata & von Leden, 1970; Kitajima & Gould, 1976; Kitajima, Tanabe & Isshiki, 1975). Orlikoff corroborated Ramig and Ringel's (1983) argument that older speakers can be differentiated by their physical status, particularly cardiovascular health.

Muscle atrophy has a significant effect on laryngeal function. Using electromyography (EMG), Ramig, Gray, Baker, Corbin-Lewis, Buder, Luschei et al. (2001) reported that older speakers demonstrate decreased EMG activity (amplitudes and firing rates) in the thyroarytenoid and lateral cricoarytenoid muscles. These changes were possibly due to muscle atrophy or reduced peripheral or central drive to the laryngeal motor neuron pool (Baker, Ramig, Luschei, & Smith, 1998; Baker, Ramig, Sapir, Luschei, & Smith, 2001; Luschei, Ramig, Baker, & Smith, 1999). In addition to these intrinsic muscular changes, Jones (1994) noted that the suspensatory musculature (elevators and depressors) also displayed decreased laryngeal elevation.

Muscular weakening within the larynx may also lead to decreased pitch range. Linville, Skarin, and Fornatto (1989) reported decreased pitch range with aging, which is likely indicative of weakening of the intrinsic muscles of the larynx, thereby reducing adduction. The result would be that air could leak through the glottis at initiation as well as demonstrating decreased upper range via weakening of the cricothyroid muscle (see discussion of glottal gaps below).

Sex plays a role in laryngeal changes as well: males and females exhibit differences in voice change with age. These changes might be best explained by the menopausal changes in women where increased vocal fold mass results in differing mechanical properties of the vocal folds (Honjo & Isshiki, 1980). In contrast, males demonstrate breathiness due to incomplete closure of the glottis and increased laryngeal tension with age, resulting in compensation for incomplete glottal closure (Ryan & Burk, 1974).

Breathiness is apparent in both younger and older female speakers; however, the source of that breathiness differs in location within the glottis (Linville, 2002). Both groups demonstrate gaps in the glottis with no significant differences in total area; however, the location of the glottal gap differs. Young women demonstrate higher spectral noise in the 3000 Hz region, indicative of a gap in the posterior region of the glottis, specifically due to separation of the arytenoids. In contrast, elderly women demonstrate higher spectral noise in the 6000 Hz range. This is due to an increased open quotient (i.e., a relatively longer open phase during vibration) and turbulent aspiration, indicative of a gap in a more anterior portion of the glottis (Linville, 1992).

Linville (2001) thought this finding was puzzling because there is sufficient evidence against posterior closure of the glottis in older speakers. The change in posterior glottal gap is indicative of a gender marker in females, and this marker is accomplished in a different way with age. In fact, increased posterior glottal adduction may be compensatory because of an inability to adequately valve in the anterior portion. Males display increased glottal gaps and demonstrate an increased open quotient with age; however, the difference between older and younger males is not significant. The change in the glottal gap of males appears to have little effect on voice.

Sapienza and Dutka (1996) reported that peak glottal air flow measures differed between elderly and young females. This finding accounts for little in predicting the age of a speaker, similar to previous work by Titze (1989) and Holmberg, Hillman, Perkell, and Guiod (1988). This contradicts Kahane (1980), who reports there is anatomical evidence to predict differences in air flow in older women, yet prior acoustic research has reported otherwise (Awan, 2006; DePinto & Hollien,

1982; Ferrand, 2002; Harnsberger, Shrivastav, Brown, Rothman, & Hollien, 2008; Higgins & Saxman, 1991; Linville & Fisher, 1985b; Mueller, Sweeney, & Baribeau, 1984; Russell, Penny, & Pemberton, 1995). Therefore, structural laryngeal changes with age may not always result in functional changes that predict a speaker's age.

Biever and Bless (1989) studied 42 females comprising two age groups. The young group had a mean age of 25 years, and the older group had a mean age of 69 years. No differences occurred between young and older female speakers on F_0, jitter, or mean air flow rate; however, older speakers demonstrated increased variability on each measure. There were significant differences in the mean shimmer and the shimmer variability between the groups. Using videostroboscopy, the authors reported that the vibratory characteristics of the vocal folds were different in older speakers (see **Table 7-1**).

Biever and Bless (1989) attributed incomplete glottal closure to decreased muscle mass and a thinning of the intermediate layer of the lamina propria. They believed that this was not a surprising finding for older female speakers. They hypothesized that the aperiodicity was due to instability of neurological control, disease-associated changes, and turbulence. However, mucosal wave changes were ascribed to edema and drying of the vocal folds as well as thinning of the superficial layer of the lamina propria, which is seen in postmenopausal women. More recent research has found evidence of neurological change in the neuromuscular system of the larynx that could lead to muscular instability, resulting in the aperiodicity described by Biever and Bless (e.g., Baker, Ramig, Luschei et al., 1998; Baker, Ramig, Sapir et al., 2001; Luschei et al., 1999; Ramig, Gray et al., 2001).

Phonation in males has also been studied. Shipp, Qi, Huntley, and Hollien (1992) examined the acoustic and temporal correlates across male speakers in the decades 20 through 90. They found that older

Table 7-1

Vibratory Characteristics of Young versus Older Females, in Descending Order of Appearance

Observation	Older Females	Younger Females
Incomplete glottal closure	90%	80%
Aperiodicity	85%	30%
Amplitude changes	50–55%	10%
Mucosal wave changes	50%	10%
Asymmetry	15%	0%
Stiffness	5%	5%

Source: Modified with permission from Biever & Bless (1989).

males had the highest F_0 in relation to middle-age and younger speakers and that these older speakers' values were significantly different from the other two groups. In addition, older speakers had longer pause times during speech units and took more breaths to complete the same productions. They also had increased utterance lengths.

Verdonck-de Leeuw and Mahieu (2004) studied age-related changes in phonation across a five-year period. The authors reported a trend toward increased F_0, a voice that was rated as more "creaky" by listeners, and self-reports of day-to-day voice changes and avoiding large parties. In addition, the voice was rated as perceptually rough with increased perturbation measures and differences in the soft phonation index. The increased soft-phonation index might reflect hypotonia of intrinsic muscles of the larynx or incomplete glottal closure.

Oropharyngeal Factors

The vocal tract also undergoes changes during the aging process. Xue and Hao (2003) studied age-related changes in the oropharyngeal structures. They looked at the changes in the length and cross-sectional diameter of the vocal tract in 38 young males and females and 38 elderly males and females. Using acoustic reflection (AR) technologies (Eccovision Acoustic Pharyngometer, Sensormedics Corp., Yorba Linda, California), they found that women and men tend to have similar patterns of vocal tract dimension changes as they age. Xue and Hao also observed that the oral cavity tends to lengthen with increased age but the pharyngeal cavity does not, and the overall vocal tract length does not increase with age. These changes may contribute to the lowering of the F1 in elderly speakers, but the authors cautioned that other factors may play a role, such as lip rounding.

Watson and Munson (2007) also described a lowering of the F1 and more back productions of mid vowels, which they did not attribute to physiological changes. Instead, they described an interaction between word frequency and vowel density (phonological nearness of neighboring words), which made for more conservative pronunciation patterns. They believed that physiological explanations of strength were not relevant because speech production operates at strength levels much below a maximum level. However, they did not measure volume changes, as did Xue and Hao (2003). Interestingly, Watson and Munson made the clear point that it is difficult to attribute all changes in articulation in older speakers to aging because societal speech patterns also change with time and that older speakers may have retained earlier articulatory strategies.

Hoit, Watson, Hixon, McMahon, and Johnson (1994) examined velopharyngeal function during speech, measuring nasal air flow across four age groups, the oldest of which was 80+ years. No age-related differences in nasal airflow were found. Their findings did not support the suggestion of Hutchinson, Robinson, and Nerbonne (1978) that velopharyngeal function deteriorates with increasing age.

Signs of Problems

Sataloff (1998) reminds us that when considering diagnosis and treatment of communication problems in the elderly, we need to consider coronary heart disease, cerebrovascular disease, hypertension, obesity, stroke, diabetes, cancer, diet, osteoporosis, hearing loss, vision loss, anemia, arthritis, neurological dysfunction including tremor, incontinence, gastrointestinal disorders, and other conditions. These conditions may influence voice and speaking in the elderly due to loss of physiological reserve.

Specific signs of presbylarynges and presbyphonia include a vocal fold bowing and prominent vocal processes during laryngeal examination, characterized as the "arrow point" (Pontes, Brasolotto, & Behlau, 2005). In addition to bowing, ventricular visibility, or prominent vocal processes, women are likely to display more edema than males, whereas the males display more vocal fold atrophy (Close & Woodson, 1989). Vocal fold bowing is due to changes in the connective tissue of the vocal folds, particularly at the deep layer of the lamina propria (Boulet & Oddens, 1996; Hirano et al., 1983; Ryan, McDonald, & Devine, 1956; Wilcox & Horii, 1980).

Overall, any breathiness that interferes with communication warrants referral to an SLP or other medical professionals. Certain vibratory characteristics also indicate that there may be a problem. Incomplete glottal closure, aperiodicity, amplitude changes, and mucosal wave changes would warrant referral to an SLP or other medical professionals. An older person with a voice that is rated as "creaky" or rough should also be seen by their physician.

Most elderly speakers are able to cope with decreased strength and flexibility of the oropharyngeal muscles and structures because the strength required for speech is much lower than the maximum strength of the oral musculature. However, one might expect the elderly person's articulatory and resonatory competence to be more fragile and that the presence of a disease process might lead to sudden breakdowns in speech capability.

Strategies to Help Older Adults' Voice and Motor Speech Abilities

The majority of older speakers in good health demonstrate typical vocal behaviors in spite of laryngeal and respiratory changes. Voice therapy might prove beneficial for those with atypical vocal behaviors.

Berg, Hapner, Klein, and Johns (2008) reported that older speakers enrolled in voice therapy, had higher voice-related quality of life measures. Patients who were more adherent to the voice therapy protocol and attended more voice therapy sessions were more likely to report improvement compared with those who were judged as "partially adherent." The adherent speakers were also more likely to see a laryngologist for reevaluation a month earlier than others.

In addition, Orlikoff's (1990) report that older speakers who are in good physical health are more likely to demonstrate vocal stability than were atherosclerotic speakers, might indicate that speakers who maintain a healthy lifestyle are more likely to avoid age-related changes in voice. This is despite the many numerous physical challenges likely to be seen in older speakers (e.g., smoking changes, environmental exposure, cerebrovascular accident).

Although voice disorders in individuals as a function of age only are rare, age-related changes in the respiratory system might make individuals less able to compensate for acquired disorders. Specifically, persons who smoke are more likely to report day-to-day changes in voice, as well as demonstrate reduced fundamental frequency, increased "creakiness," perceptually rough voice, and increased frequency perturbation (jitter) (Verdonck-Leeuw & Mahieu, 2004). Strategies that emphasize increased muscle activity, such as pulling and pushing, are probably not appropriate, as they could result in hyperfunctional behavior. Rather, strategies that optimize vocal function itself (i.e., Vocal Function Exercises or Resonant Voice Therapy), are more likely to lead to a better voice without hyperfunction.

Instrumentation and Evaluation

The differences in speakers across the age range are numerous, and many clinical tools are available for assessment, for assistance in interpretation, and for providing documentation and feedback during treatment. Even though modern equipment is impressive in its capability and reliability, the data collected during a speech and voice assessment are only as valid and reliable as the individual collecting them. Many variables must be taken into account when collecting these data. For instance, intensity measurements require a constant microphone-to-mouth distance, best provided by a head-mounted microphone. A hand-held microphone allows for movement either toward or away from the source and provides data that, while objective, are difficult to interpret or are unusable. The necessary steps to ensure appropriate data collection are outside the scope of this chapter; however, there are many useful texts available to SLPs that introduce the collection of objective measurements to clinicians and scientists alike (e.g., Baken &

Orlikoff, 2000). The importance of using standard procedures in data collection cannot be overstated. Comparisons to previous research and normative data are not possible without maintaining standard protocols and procedures.

Perceptual Ratings

Perceptual ratings of voice and disorder severity are dependent upon the training and experience of the clinician as well as the validity of the scale used. Consequently, it is difficult to establish high reliability of perceptual ratings of voice across clinicians and clinical settings. There are numerous ratings scales available to clinicians, with each providing different opportunities for measurement and varying reliability and validity. The GRBAS scale (Hirano, 1981) has long been used to rate the following: Grade, Roughness, Breathiness, Asthenia, and Strain. However, the agreement among raters is reliable only at the extremes. The severely disordered and normal voices are reliably rated, but voices that are mild-moderate and moderate-severe are less likely to be rated similarly across clinicians (DeKrom, 1994). In addition, listeners across languages are not reliable in their ratings within the individual categories (Yamaguchi, Shrivastav, Andrews, & Nimi, 2003). Recently, the Consensus Auditory Perceptual Evaluation of Voice (CAPE-V; ASHA, 2003) has been developed to better standardize the perceptual ratings associated with expert clinicians' evaluations.

In addition to perceptual ratings by clinicians, there are instruments designed for patients to indicate the severity of their voice problems and the effect that the voice disturbance has on their life. Instruments of note include the voice-related quality of life (VRQOL; Hogikyan & Sethuraman, 1999) and the voice handicap index (VHI; Jacobson, Johnson, Grywalski, & Silbergleit, 1977). Karnell, Melton, Childes, Coleman, Dailey, and Hoffman (2007) reported that the standard ratings systems of the GRBAS and CAPE-V were comparable in reliably describing a voice problem; however, patient-reported rating scales were not strongly correlated to perceptual measures of voice. This information provides another example that corroborates clinicians' reports of instances where client perception and clinician perception are dissimilar.

Videostroboscopic

Videostroboscopic evaluation is often considered the gold standard for evaluating voice disorders by allowing visualization of the larynx and true vocal folds. However, it is essential to remember that videostroboscopy is a *subjective* tool in the overall evaluation of voice. The KayPentax Digital Video Stroboscopy System, Model 9295 (KayPentax; Lincoln Park, New Jersey) is the latest in the line of videostroboscopy units in use since the early 1990s. The most recent unit allows for digital storage of examinations and provides a patient database and acoustic analysis software. The Lx Strobe3 (Laryngograph; London, United Kingdom) provides many of the same features. Each of these products provides images that can be saved and interpreted at a later time and are useful for pre- and post-treatment comparisons. Indirect laryngoscopy can be completed using rigid or flexible laryngeal scopes. The flexible scope allows visualization of the larynx in more "typical" activity during voice production compared to the rigid scope that requires the clinician to hold the tongue and the client to open the mouth widely. Consequently, each technique has advantages and disadvantages. Flexible endoscopy can be used with all ages and is especially useful with those individuals who have overly active gag reflexes. A major advantage of flexible endoscopy is that the patient is able to speak, sing, exercise (limited), and swallow. A major disadvantage is that the quality of the image is poorer than that obtained with a rigid endoscope for brightness and magnification of the image. Since more light can be brought to bear on the vocal folds with rigid endoscopy, the rigid scope is particularly useful for documenting the mucosal wave, structural integrity of the vocal fold (e.g., identifying sulcus vocalis), and other biomechanics of vocal fold vibration.

Acoustic

The KayPentax Computerized Speech Lab (CSL) is a dedicated hardware and software platform that provides a comprehensive system for speech and voice analyses. This system includes a number of add-on programs that comprehensively address differing acoustic aspects of voice and speech. In particular, the CSL provides a disordered voice database that has extensive normative data on acoustic measures associated with typical and disordered voices. KayPentax Sona-Speech II and Multi-Speech can be installed on a laptop computer, allowing greater portability while including most of the analysis features of the CSL. Laryngograph produces similar products, such as Speech Studio, which allows for connecting to a laptop computer via a standard USB cable. In addition WEVOSYS (Frocheim, Germany) has many software programs (e.g., their lingWAVES line) available for use in a voice clinic. The products include all necessary measures for an adequate evaluation and include normative data across the life span.

Physiologic Measures

KayPentax has recently released the Phonatory Aerodynamic System (PAS). The PAS allows clinicians to collect data important to an overall voice assessment of average phonatory flow rate, sound pressure level, fundamental frequency, vital capacity, subglottal pressure (derived), glottal resistance, and efficiency parameters; however, established normative data using the PAS are not yet available. The Glottal Enterprises Aeroview system (Syracuse, New York) allows for data collection similar to the PAS and is easily transferred from desktop to desktop or laptop and requires no dedicated hardware configurations.

There are a number of exceptional software programs available to clinicians in addition to those mentioned from KayPentax and Glottal Enterprises. The TF32, time-frequency analysis software program for 32-bit Windows (Milenkovic, 2002), is a program that allows for acoustic and aerodynamic data collection. For example, the standard program measures intensity, frequency, spectrograms, jitter, shimmer, and signal-to-noise ratio. The program can also be tailored to the needs of the clinic. The program does require the purchase of other hardware, particularly aerodynamic equipment, microphones, and sound cards. This program does not provide normative data with purchase but is a powerful tool in the hands of a clinician that has access to, and can adequately interpret, normative data.

Velopharyngeal Evaluation

SLPs have numerous hardware and software choices available for assessment of velopharyngeal (VP) function. The Nasometer II (KayPentax) allows for comparisons of oral and nasal acoustic energy via two microphones separated by a plate under the speaker's nose. This system is well established as a tool in speech and voice sciences and has exceptional validity. The system is equipped with standard reading passages as well as the Simplified Nasometric Assessment Procedures (SNAP) test (syllable repetition/prolonged sounds, picture-cued subtests, and reading; Kummer, 2008) for use with children. The normative data for the SNAP test are for pediatric patients. The acoustic signals derived from the system are noted by the manufacturer to correlate well with aerodynamic measures of VP function. However, these acoustic signals cannot replace the physiologic measures available in systems previously mentioned (PAS, TF32, Glottal Enterprises). The Nasality Visualization System by Glottal Enterprises combines the acoustic information in addition to nasal and oral pressures. The system allows for auditory feedback for the patient, as well as providing visual feedback representing nasality. This is a tool that is appropriate for hypernasality as a result of motor speech disorders and cleft palate/craniofacial disorders.

In summary, there are many diagnostic tools available to SLPs in the evaluation of voice and motor speech abilities in older adults.

However, there is a need for standardization of procedures across clinicians and clinical settings. Many hardware and software configurations have been mentioned in this chapter, but only a small number of them have normative data available. In essence, the equipment mentioned is only as good as the professional operating it and requires the diligence of the clinician and scientist to seek out the appropriate normative data from the research. It is then that clinicians can apply normative data in their interpretation of patient performance.

Quick Facts

- General Changes in Voice and Motor Speech of Neurologically Intact Older Adults:
  - Changes include diminished volume, breathiness, possible increases in pitch, diminished flexibility, and tremulousness
  - Fundamental frequency (F_0) decreases with maturity and then increases in older age
  - Phonatory stability decreases
  - Older adults have diminished pitch ranges and maximum phonation times
  - Variability of vocal production (shimmer and jitter) may increase with age
  - Descriptions of changes in voice and speech specific to aging are rare
  - Diagnosis of age-related changes should be made with caution so as not to miss a primary diagnosis masquerading as an age-related change
- Factors That Can Negatively Affect Older Adults' Voice and Motor Speech Abilities:
  - Respiratory factors:
    - Increased stiffness of the respiratory system and weaker respiratory muscles are common with increasing age
    - Elastic recoil of respiratory structures decreases related to calcification of the costal and rib/vertebral articulations
    - Osteoporosis of the vertebrae can lead to dorsal kyphosis ("hunchback") and increased anterior-posterior dimension of the chest wall ("barrel chest")
    - Loss of elasticity in the pleural membrane
    - Loss of recoil, which leads to speaking at higher lung volumes

- ○ Reduced muscle strength, which makes compensation difficult or impossible to maintain when other challenges are present
- ○ Increase in residual volume and functional residual capacity
- ○ Decreases in muscular force due to:
  - ❏ Nutritional status or weight
  - ❏ Decreased muscle mass, both cross-sectional muscle fiber and the number of muscle fibers
  - ❏ Reduced type II or "fast twitch fibers"
  - ❏ Altered neuromuscular junction
  - ❏ Denervated muscle fibers, specifically type II
- ○ Peripheral airways lose support and tend to narrow
- ○ Terminal air spaces remain open, thus, trapping air
- ○ Decrease in number of alveoli
- ○ Decreased sensitivity to conditions of hypercapnia and hypoxia
- ○ Asthma
- ■ Laryngeal factors:
  - ○ Muscle atrophy
  - ○ Gender
    - ❏ Menopausal changes lead to increase vocal fold mass, which results in differing mechanical properties of the vocal folds
    - ❏ Males demonstrate breathiness due to incomplete closure of the glottis and increased laryngeal tension
    - ❏ Glottal gaps appear in both men and women, with the total glottal gap area about equal
    - ❏ For young women, there is more often a posterior gap with lower spectral noise, and for older women, there is more often an anterior gap with higher spectral noise
    - ❏ For men, there are no significant changes in the location and size of gap
    - ❏ Postmenopausal changes such as edema and drying of the vocal folds lead to mucosal wave changes
    - ❏ Phonation changes in males include increased F_0, longer pause times during speech, and increased utterance lengths
- ■ Oropharyngeal factors:
  - ○ Women and men tend to have similar patterns of vocal tract dimension changes as they age

- ○ Oral cavity lengthens with age, but the pharyngeal cavity and overall length of the vocal tract do not change; lower F1 may result
  - ○ Velopharyngeal function does not appear to change with age
- Signs That an Older Adult Should Be Referred to a Speech-Language Pathologist or Other Medical Professionals
  - Presence of breathiness interfering with communication
  - Signs of presbylarynges and presbyphonia: vocal fold bowing, prominent vocal processes characterized as the "arrow point," and ventricular visibility
  - Vibratory characteristics including:
    - ○ Incomplete glottal closure
    - ○ Aperiodicity
    - ○ Amplitude changes
    - ○ Mucosal wave changes
  - Voice is rated as "creaky" or rough, patient reports of day-to-day voice changes or avoiding social gatherings such as large parties
  - Sudden breakdowns in speech capability
- Strategies That Can Help Older Adults Voice and Motor Speech Abilities:
  - Participation in voice therapy and learning strategies that optimize vocal function such as Vocal Function Exercises or Resonant Voice Therapy
  - Staying in good health
  - Not smoking
  - *Avoiding* strategies that emphasize increased muscle activity, such as pulling and pushing to increase closure, because they can result in hyperfunctional behavior
- Instrumentation and Evaluation:
  - Perceptual ratings of voice and disorder severity depend upon training and experience of the clinician and the validity of the scale used
  - Perceptual ratings instruments include the GRBAS, the Consensus Auditory Perceptual Evaluation of Voice, the voice-related quality of life, and the voice handicap index
  - Videostroboscopic evaluation is considered the gold standard for evaluating voice disorders, but it is subjective in nature
  - Videostroboscopic evaluation options include flexible and rigid endoscopy
  - Tools for acoustic measures include the Computerized Speech Lab, Sona-Speech II, Multi-Speech, Laryngograph, Time-Frequency Analysis 32-bit, and WEVOSYS

- Instruments for physiologic measures include the Phonatory Aerodynamic System and the Aeroview System
- The Nasometer II and the Nasality Visualization System can be used to evaluate velopharyngeal function
- Although many diagnostic tools are available, there is a lack of standardization of procedures across clinicians and clinical settings

Discussion Questions

1. Is there a specific age when fundamental frequency begins to increase?
2. What could contribute to older adults having a "creaky" voice quality?
3. What vocal characteristics do you associate with aging?
4. Are there any hormonal influences involved in age-related voice changes in men and women?

References

American Speech-Language-Hearing Association (2003). CAPE-V; Consensus Auditory-Perceptual Evaluation of Voice. Rockville, MD: Division 2.

Arora N. S., & Rochester, D. F. (1982). Respiratory muscle strength and maximal voluntary ventilation in undernourished patients. *American Review of Respiratory Disease*, 126, 5–8.

Awan, S. N. (2006). The aging female voice: Acoustic and respiratory data. *Clinical Linguistics and Phonetics*, 20, 171–180.

Ayres, J. G. (1990). Late onset asthma. *British Medical Journal*, 300, 1602–1603.

Baken, R. J. (2005). The aged voice: A new hypothesis. *Journal of Voice*, 19, 317–325.

Baken, R. J., & Orlikoff, R. F. (2000). *Clinical measurement of speech and voice* (2nd ed.). San Diego, CA: Singular Publishing.

Baker, K. K., Ramig, L. O., Luschei, E. S., & Smith, M. E. (1998). Thyroarytenoid muscle activity associated with hypophonia in Parkinson disease and aging. *Neurology*, 51, 1592–1598.

Baker, K. K., Ramig, L. O., Sapir, S., Luschei, E. S., & Smith, M. E. (2001). Control of vocal loudness in young and old adults. *Journal of Speech, Language, and Hearing Research*, 44, 297–305.

Bassey, E. J., & Harries, U. J. (1993). Normal values for handgrip strength in 920 men and women aged over 65 years, and longitudinal changes over 4 years in 620 survivors. *Clinical Science*, 84, 331–337.

Benjamin, B. J. (1981). Frequency variability in the aged voice. *Journal of Gerontology*, 36, 722–726.

Berg, E. E., Hapner, E., Klein, A., & Johns, M. M., III. (2008). Voice therapy improves quality of life in age-related dysphonia: A case-control study. *Journal of Voice*, 22, 70–74.

Biever, D., & Bless, D. (1989). Vibratory characteristics of the vocal folds of young adult and geriatric women. *Journal of Voice*, 3, 120–131.

Boulet, M. J., & Oddens, B. J. (1996). Female voice changes around and after the menopause: An initial investigation. *Maturitas*, 23, 15–21.

Brown, M., & Hasser, E. (1996). Complexity of age-related change in skeletal muscle. *Journals of Gerontology Series A: Biological Sciences and Medical Sciences*, 51, 117–123.

Brown, W., Morris, R., & Michel, J. (1989). Vocal jitter in young adult and aged female voices. *Journal of Voice*, 3, 113–119.

Burrows, B., Cline, M. G., Knudson, R. J., Taussig, L. M., & Lebowitz, M. D. (1983). A descriptive analysis of the growth and decline of the FVC and FEV1. *Chest*, 83, 717–724.

Chan, E. D., & Welsh, C. H. (1998). Geriatric respiratory medicine. *Chest*, 114, 1704–1733.

Close, L. G., & Woodson, G. E. (1989). Common upper airway disorders in the elderly and their management. *Geriatrics*, 44, 67–71.

Crapo, R. O. (1993). The aging lung. In D. A. Mahler (Ed.), *Pulmonary disease in the elderly patient* (vol. 63, pp. 1–21). New York: Marcel Dekker.

Davis, S. B. (1979). Acoustic characteristics of normal and pathological voices. In N. J. Lass (Ed.), *Speech and language: Advances in basic research and practice* (vol. 1, pp. 271–335). New York: Academic Press.

DeKrom, G. (1994). Consistency and reliability of voice quality ratings for different types of speech fragments. *Journal of Speech and Hearing Research*, 37, 985–1000.

De Pinto, O., & Hollien, H. (1982). Speaking fundamental frequency characteristics of Australian women: Then and now. *Journal of Phonetics*, 10, 367–375.

Dhar, S., Shastri, S. R., & Lenora, R. A. K. (1976). Aging and the respiratory system. *Medical Clinics of North America*, 60, 1121–1139.

Enright, P. L., Kronmal, R. A., Manolio, T. A., Schenker, M. B., & Hyatt, R. E. (1994). Respiratory muscle strength in the elderly: Correlates and reference values. *American Journal of Respiratory and Critical Care Medicine*, 149, 430–438.

Evans, R., Mullally, D. I., Wilson, R. W., Gergen, P. J., Rosenberg, H. M., Grauman, J. S. et al., (1987). National trends in the morbidity and mortality of asthma in the US: Prevalence, hospitalization, and death from asthma over two decades: 1965–1984. *Chest*, 91, 65S–74S.

Ferrand, C. (2002). Harmonics-to-noise ratio: An index of vocal aging. *Journal of Voice*, 16, 480–487.

Glottal Enterprises. *Glottal Enterprises Aeroview System*. Syracuse, NY: author.

Gorham-Rowan, M. M., & Laures-Gore, J. (2006). Acoustic-perceptual correlates of voice quality in elderly men and women. *Journal of Communication Disorders*, 39, 171–184.

Harnsberger, J. D., Shrivastav, R., Brown, W. S., Jr., Rothman, H., & Hollien, H. (2008). Speaking rate and fundamental frequency as cues to perceived age in speech. *Journal of Voice*, 22, 58–69.

Higgins, M. B., & Saxman, J. H. (1991). A comparison of selected phonatory behaviors of healthy aged and young adults. *Journal of Speech and Hearing Research*, 34, 1000–1010.

Hirano, M. (1981). *Clinical examination of voice*. New York: Springer-Verlag.

Hirano, M., Kurita, S., & Nakashima, T. (1983). Growth, development and aging of human vocal fold. In D. M. Bless and J. H. Abbs (Eds.), *Vocal fold physiology* (pp. 22–43). San Diego, CA: College-Hill.

Hixon, T. J., Goldman, M. D., & Mead, J. (1973). Kinematics of the chest wall during speech production: Volume displacements of the rib cage, abdomen, and lung. *Journal of Speech and Hearing Research*, 16, 78–115.

Hixon, T. J., Mead, J., & Goldman, M. D. (1976). Dynamics of the chest wall during speech production: Function of the thorax, rib cage, diaphragm, and abdomen. *Journal of Speech and Hearing Research*, 19, 297–356.

Hogikyan, N. D., & Sethuraman, G. (1999). Validation of an instrument to measure voice-related quality of life (V-RQOL). *Journal of Voice*, 13, 557–569.

Hoit, J. D., & Hixon, T. J. (1987). Age and speech breathing. *Journal of Speech and Hearing Research*, 30, 351–366.

Hoit, J. D., Hixon, T. J., Altman, M. E., & Morgan, W. J. (1989). Speech breathing in women. *Journal of Speech and Hearing Research*, 32, 353–365.

Hoit, J., Watson, P., Hixon, K., McMahon, P., & Johnson, C. (1994). Age and velopharyngeal function during speech production. *Journal of Speech and Hearing Research*, 37, 295–302.

Holmberg, E. B., Hillman, R. E., Perkell, J. S., & Guiod, P. C. (1988). Comparisons among aerodynamic, electroglottographic, and acoustic spectral measures of female voice. *Journal of Speech and Hearing Research*, 38, 1212–1223.

Honjo, I., & Isshiki, N. (1980). Laryngoscopic and voice characteristics of aged persons. *Archives of Otolaryngology*, 106, 149–150.

Hutchinson, J., Robinson, K., & Nerbonne, M. (1978). Patterns of nasalance in a sample of normal gerontologic subjects. *Journal of Communication Disorders*, 11, 469–481.

Iwata, S. (1972). Periodicities of perturbations in normal and pathologic larynges. *Laryngoscope*, 82, 87–95.

Iwata, S., & von Leden, H. (1970). Pitch perturbations in normal and pathological voices. *Folia Phoniatrica*, 22, 413–424.

Jacobson, B., Johnson, A., Grywalski, C., & Silbergleit, A. (1977). The voice handicap index (VHI): Development and validation. *American Journal of Speech Language Pathology*, 6, 66–70.

Janssens, J. P., Pache, J. C., & Nicod, L. P. (1999). Physiological changes in respiratory function associated with ageing. *European Respiratory Journal*, 13, 197–205.

Jones, B. (1994). The pharynx: Disorders of function. *Radiologic Clinics of North America*, 32, 1103–1115.

Kahane, J. C. (1980). Age-related histological changes in the human male and female laryngeal cartilages: Biological and functional implications. In V. Lawrence (Ed.), *Transcripts of the Ninth Symposium: Care of the Professional Voice*. New York: The Voice Foundation.

Kahane, J. C. (1981). Changes in the aging peripheral speech mechanism. In D. S. Beasley & G. A. Davis (Eds.), *Aging: Communication processes and disorders*. New York: Grune & Stratton.

Kahane, J. C. (1983). A survey of age-related changes in the connected tissues of the adult human larynx. In D. Bless & J. Abbs (Eds.), *Vocal physiology*. San Diego, CA: College Hill Press.

Kahane, J. (1987). Connective tissue changes in the larynx and their effects on voice. *Journal of Voice*, 1, 27–30.

Kahane, J. (1988). Age related changes in the human cricoarytenoid joint. In O. Fujimara (Ed.), *Vocal physiology: Voice production, mechanisms, and functions*. New York: Raven.

Kahane, J. (1990). Age-related changes in the peripheral speech mechanism: Structural and physiological changes. In E. Cherow (Ed.), *Proceedings of the Research Symposium on Communication Skills and Aging* (pp. 75–87). Rockville, MD: American Speech-Language-Hearing Association.

Karnell, M. P., Melton, S. D., Childes, J. M., Coleman, T. C., Dailey, S. A., & Hoffman, H. T. (2007). Reliability of clinician-based (GRBAS and CAPE-V) and patient-based (V-RQOL and IPVI) documentation of voice disorders. *Journal of Voice*, 21 (5), 576–590.

Kay Pentax (2008). *Digital video stroboscopy system; Model 9295*. Retrieved from http://www.kayelemetrics.com/Product%20Info/Strobe%20Systems/9295.htm

Kendall, K. (2007). Presbyphonia: A review. *Current Opinion in Otolaryngology and Head and Neck Surgery*, 15, 137–140.

Kitajima, K., & Gould, W. J. (1976). Vocal shimmer in sustained phonation of normal and pathologic voice. *Annals of Otolaryngology*, 85, 377–381.

Kitajima, K., Tanabe, M., & Isshiki, N. (1975). Pitch perturbation in normal and pathological voice. *Studia Phonologica*, 9, 25–32.

Kummer, A. W. (2008). *Cleft palate and craniofacial anomalies: Effects on speech and resonance* (2nd ed.). San Diego, CA: Singular.

Laryngograph. LxStrobe3 digital precision stroboscopy. Retrieved from http://www.laryngograph.com/pr_lxstrobe.htm on December 1, 2009.

Lexell, J. (1997). Evidence for nervous system degeneration with advancing age. *Journal of Nutrition, 5 Suppl.t,* 1011S–1013S.

Linville, S. (1992). Glottal configurations in two age groups of women. *Journal of Speech and Hearing Research,* 35, 1209–1215.

Linville, S. E. (2001). *Vocal aging.* San Diego, CA: Singular Publishing Group.

Linville, S. (2002). Source characteristics of aged voice assessed from long-term average spectra. *Journal of Voice,* 16, 472–479.

Linville, S., & Fisher, H. (1985a). Acoustic characteristics of perceived versus actual age in controlled phonation by adult females. *Journal of the Acoustical Society of America,* 78, 40–48.

Linville, S., & Fisher, H. (1985b). Acoustic characteristics of women's voices with advancing age. *Journal of Gerontology,* 40, 324–330.

Linville, S. E., & Korabic, E. W. (1986). Elderly listeners' estimates of vocal age in adult females. *Journal of the Acoustical Society of America,* 80, 692–694.

Linville, S. E., Skarin, B. D., & Fornatto, E. (1989). The interrelationship of measures related to vocal function, speech rate, and laryngeal appearance in elderly women. *Journal of Speech and Hearing Research,* 32, 323–330.

Luschei, E. S., Ramig, L. O., Baker, K. L., & Smith, M. E. (1999). Discharge characteristics of laryngeal single motor units during phonation in young and older adults and in persons with Parkinson disease. *Journal of Neurophysiology,* 81, 2121–2139.

McGlone, R., & Hollien, H. (1963). Vocal pitch characteristics of aged women. *Journal of Speech and Hearing Research,* 6, 164–170.

McKeown, F. (1965). *Pathology of the aged.* London: Butterworths.

Meyer, K. C. (2005). Aging. *Proceedings of the American Thoracic Society,* 2, 433–439.

Milenkovic, P. (2002). *TF32 time frequency analysis software program for 32-bit Windows* [Computer software]. Madison, WI: author.

Moorman, J. E., & Mannino, D. M. (2001). Increasing U. S. asthma mortality rates: Who is really dying? *Journal of Asthma,* 38, 65–71.

Mueller, P. B., Sweeney, R. J., & Baribeau, L. J. (1984). Acoustic and morphologic study of the senescent voice. *Ear, Nose, and Throat Journal,* 63, 71–75.

Murray, J. F. (1986). Aging. In J. F. Murray (Ed.), *The normal lung.* Philadelphia: W. B. Saunders.

Orlikoff, R. (1990). The relationship between age and cardiovascular health to certain acoustic characteristics of male voices. *Journal of Speech and Hearing Research,* 33, 450–457.

Pierce, J. A., & Ebert, R. V. (1965). Fibrous network of the lung and its change with age. *Thorax,* 20, 469–476.

Polkey, M. I., Harris, M. L., Hughes, P. D., Hamengard, C. H., Lyons, D., & Moxham, J. (1997). The contractile properties of the elderly human diaphragm. *American Journal of Respiratory and Critical Care Medicine,* 155, 1560–1564.

Pontes, P., Brasolotto, A., & Behlau, M. (2005). Glottic characteristics and voice complaint in the elderly. *Journal of Voice,* 19, 84–94.

Ptacek, P., & Sander, E. (1966). Age recognition from voice. *Journal of Speech and Hearing Research,* 9, 273–277.

Ptacek, P., Sander, E., Maloney, W., & Jackson, C. (1966). Phonatory and related changes with advanced age. *Journal of Speech and Hearing Research,* 9, 353–360.

Ramig, L. O., Gray, S., Baker, K., Corbin-Lewis, K., Buder, E., Luschei, E., et al. (2001). The aging voice: A review, treatment data, and familial and genetic perspectives. *Folia Phoniatrica et Logopaedica,* 53, 252–265.

Ramig, L., & Ringel, R. (1983). Effects of physiological aging on selected acoustic characteristics of voice. *Journal of Speech and Hearing Research, 26*, 22–30.

Robin, E. D. (1988). Risk benefit analysis in chest medicine: Death from bronchial asthma. *Chest, 93*, 614–618.

Russell, A., Penny, L., & Pemberton, C. (1995). Speaking fundamental frequencychanges over time in women: A longitudinal study. *Journal of Speech and Hearing Research, 38*, 101–109.

Ryan, R. F., McDonald, J. R., & Devine, K. D. (1956). Changes in laryngeal epithelium: Relation to age, sex, and certain other factors. *Mayo Clinic Proceedings, 31*, 47–52.

Ryan, W., & Burk, K. (1974). Perceptual and acoustic correlates in the speech of males. *Journal of Communication Disorders, 7*, 181–192.

Sapienza, C., & Dutka, J. (1996). Glottal airflow characteristics of women's voice production along an aging continuum. *Journal of Speech and Hearing Research, 39*, 322–328.

Sataloff, R. T. (1998). *Vocal health and pedagogy*. San Diego, CA: Singular.

Sataloff, R. T., Rosen, D. C., Hawkshaw, M., & Spiegel, J. R. (1997). The aging adult voice. *Journal of Voice, 11*, 156–160.

Shipp, T., & Hollien, H. (1969). Perception of the aging male voice. *Journal of Speech and Hearing Research, 12*, 703–712.

Shipp, T., Qi, Y., Huntley, R., & Hollien, H. (1992). Acoustic and temporal correlates of perceived age. *Journal of Voice, 6*, 211–216.

Sly, R. M. (1984). Increases in deaths from asthma. *Annals of Allergy, 53*, 20–25.

Sperry, E. E., & Klich, R. J. (1992). Speech breathing in senescent and younger women during oral reading. *Journal of Speech and Hearing Research, 35*, 1246–1255.

Titze, I. R. (1989). Physiologic and acoustic differences between male and female voices. *Journal of the Acoustical Society of America, 85*, 1699–1707.

Tolep, K., Higgins, N., Muza, S., Criner, G., & Kelsen, S. (1995). Comparison of diaphragm strength between healthy adult elderly and young men. *American Journal of Respiratory and Critical Care Medicine, 152*, 677–682.

Tolep, K., & Kelsen, S. (1993). Effect of aging on respiratory skeletal muscles. *Clinics in Chest Medicine, 14*, 363–378.

Verbeken, E., Cauberghs, M., & Mertens, I. (1992). The senile lung. Comparison with normal and emphysematous lungs. I: Structural aspects. *Chest, 101*, 793–799.

Verdonck-de Leeuw, I. M., & Mahieu, H. F. (2004). Vocal aging and the impact on daily life: A longitudinal study. *Journal of Voice, 18*, 193–202.

Watson, P. J. & Munson, B. (2007). A comparison of vowel acoustics in older and younger adults. *International Congress of Phonetic Sciences, 16*, 561–564.

WEVOSYS, Forcheim, Germany. http://www.wevosys.com

Wilcox, K., & Horii, Y. (1980). Age and changes in vocal jitter. *Journal of Gerontology, 35*, 194–198.

Woo, P., Casper, J., Colton, R., & Brewer, D. (1992). Dysphonia in the aging: Physiology versus disease. *Laryngoscope, 102*, 139–144.

Xue, S. A., & Hao, G. J. (2003). Changes in the human vocal tract due to aging and the acoustic correlates of speech production: A pilot study. *Journal of Speech, Language and Hearing Research, 46*, 689–701.

Yamaguchi, H., Shrivastav, R., Andrews, M. L., & Niimi, S. (2003). A comparison of voice quality ratings made by Japanese and American listeners using the GRBAS scale. *Folia Phoniatrica et Logopedia, 55* (3), 115–127.

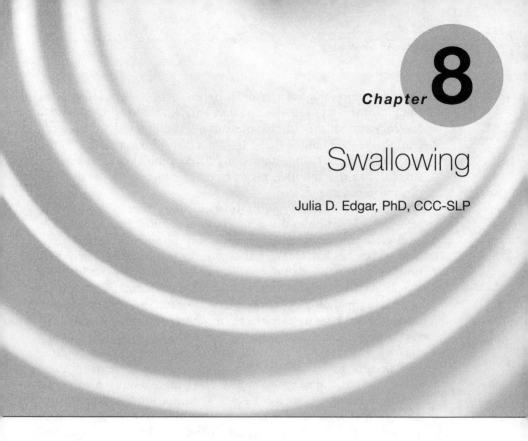

Julia D. Edgar, PhD, CCC-SLP

Swallowing

Introduction

Terms associated with eating, such as *mealtime, food,* and *drink,* bring to mind myriad associations, including socialization, nutrition, and comfort. As we anticipate a meal, we often look forward to the company of friends and/or family. Our senses are bombarded by the aroma of the food as it is prepared, followed by the visual presentation of a meal. With anticipation of the first mouthful, salivation begins, and with initial presentation of food to the mouth, the physical act of swallowing is initiated. But as we savor the textures and tastes of our meal, there is typically little thought given to the anatomical and physiological underpinnings of swallowing. Even less thought is directed toward the mature, adult swallow as it degrades over time. Clinicians and researchers have determined that the normal swallow gradually deteriorates as an adult ages. These alterations in swallowing are referred to as *presbyglutition,* or "old swallow." Like other aspects of aging, presbyglutition is more closely associated with biological age than with chronological age, and progression of biological age varies significantly from one person to the next, contributing to the overall heterogeneity of the elderly population. In addition, there are problems that are not limited to the aged, but that seem to manifest in that population more than in the young. These problems, such as xerostomia (i.e., dry mouth), may further complicate the swallowing process in older adults.

Research on presbyglutition has focused primarily on a well-screened population so that comorbidities commonly found in older adults are not represented in the study population. From these data we know that older adults with no comorbidities may have presbyglutition, but will not have dysphagia (difficulty swallowing). Dysphagia itself is not a disease but rather a symptom of one or more underlying pathologies (Groher & Bukatman, 1986). Neurological disorders and head/neck cancers are well-known causes of dysphagia. However, little to no information exists on dysphagia in older persons who have non-neurological or noncancerous comorbidities such as diabetes, congestive heart failure, or other ailments common to older adults (Kuhlemeier, 1994). Thus, presbyglutition will deteriorate to dysphagia in some elderly but not others. Although the older patient with comorbidities is more likely to develop problems swallowing, the ambiguity of when and in whom dysphagia will manifest makes it difficult to anticipate and recognize the problem. To further obscure the diagnosis of dysphagia in this population, many older adults present with complex medical profiles, and the insidious onset of dysphagia associated with aging may well be overshadowed by other, more overt, medical issues. As a result of the disparity in the age-swallow relationship, older community-dwelling persons and their family members, along with many healthcare providers, do not anticipate the potential deterioration in swallowing ability and are therefore less likely to monitor for changes in swallowing function. Even when individuals start to experience difficulty swallowing, they may associate it with the natural aging process and not mention it to their physician (Bloem et al., 1990). Consequently, they remain unaware of diagnostic tests and available treatments. Herein lies a primary reason for speech-language pathologists to gain familiarity with some of the changes inherent in the aging swallow.

This chapter will discuss what aging adults' swallowing abilities generally should be, factors that can negatively affect older adults' swallowing, signs that may warrant referral to a speech-language pathologist or other medical professionals, and what strategies can help aging adults with swallowing difficulties. A list of "Quick Facts" at the end of the chapter summarizes important points.

Older Adults' General Swallowing Abilities

Terminology associated with the medical model of screening (Goldberg & Wittes, 1981) can be used to describe the change from a young, healthy swallow to an aging swallow (presbyglutition), to a disordered swallow (dysphagia). A young adult swallow represents the *normal* state. Characteristics of a young adult swallow serve as the point of comparison for alterations in swallowing function, whether from aging or disease. Research indicates that aging changes may begin as early as age 45. These age-associated alterations in the anatomical and physiological underpinnings of deglutition, biologically present but asymptomatic and undetectable by current medical technology, represent the *latent* state. As changes progress they become detectable by specialized testing methods but remain asymptomatic, thus entering a *preclinical* state. The preclinical state is reflected in much of the literature on aging changes in healthy older adults. Study participants in this body of research are generally screened to represent characteristics of presbyglutition without contamination by illnesses or conditions that might also promote changes in swallowing. Initially, these changes in swallowing are unlikely to interfere with functional nutrition or hydration. However, there is a point of deterioration where cumulative changes of presbyglutition transition to dysphagia, even without a specific medical condition. The emergence of the *clinical* state is reached when dysphagia is symptomatic and detectable by routine care.

Normal Swallowing in the Healthy, Young Adult: A Foundation for Comparison

Adult swallowing physiology is typically described as having three discrete phases, even though in reality swallowing is a dynamic and overlapping process. The oral, pharyngeal, and esophageal phases make up the overall swallow. The oral phase is subdivided into oral preparation and oral transport. Oral preparation of food and liquid is of variable duration depending on bite or swallow size, temperature, texture, and taste. Oral preparation of solid foods requires mastication (chewing), salivary lubrication, and tongue movement. The softened mass of chewed food (bolus) is transported through the oral cavity to the pharynx via the central groove in the tongue. Liquids do not require oral preparation and are transported immediately to the pharynx via the central groove of the tongue. Duration of oral transport is approximately one second.

Timing and overlapping mechanics of the pharyngeal phase are well orchestrated to ensure that food and liquid are directed to the stomach and not the airway or the nasal passages. Six critical components make up the pharyngeal phase (Logemann, 1998): (1) elevation and retraction of the soft palate for complete closure of the velopharyngeal port; (2) superior and anterior movement of the hyoid bone and larynx; (3) laryngeal closure and cessation of breathing; (4) opening of the cricopharyngeal sphincter; (5) ramping of the tongue base; and (6) contraction from top to bottom of the pharyngeal constrictors. Duration of the pharyngeal phase is approximately one second.

The esophageal phase begins when the bolus first passes through the cricopharyngeal sphincter and ends when the bolus enters the stomach through the lower esophageal sphincter. Duration of the esophageal phase is from 8 to 20 seconds.

The Latent State of Presbyglutition: Biology of Age-Related Swallowing Decline

Many changes in the underlying anatomy and physiology of swallowing in aging humans have been documented. Nervous system changes include decreased nerve conduction velocities as well as reduced neurotransmitter levels (Weismer & Liss, 1991). Atrophy and fibrosis of muscle associated with aging result in reduced range, speed, and accuracy of structural movement. For example, differentially altered muscle-fiber type composition has been noted in the human lateral pterygoid, a muscle involved in mouth opening, and the digastric muscle, a muscle involved in mouth opening and elevation of the hyoid bone (Monemi, Liu, Thornell, & Eriksson, 2000). Fat content in the tongue increases approximately 2.7% per decade, possibly contributing to sarcopenia (i.e., age-related loss of muscle mass and strength) in the tongue (Rother, Wohlgemuth, Wolff, & Rebentrost, 2002). Laryngeal age-related changes are also noteworthy. Reduced motor unit firing rate (Luschei, Ramig, Baker, & Smith, 1999; Takeda, Thomas, & Ludlow, 2000), atrophy and loss of laryngeal muscle fibers (Malmgren, Fisher, Jones, Bookman, & Uno, 2000), ossification of laryngeal cartilage (Casiano, Ruiz, & Goldstein, 1994), increased irregularity of the laryngeal cartilage articular surfaces (Casiano et al., 1994; Kahn & Kahane, 1986), and reduced sensation in the pharynx and larynx (Aviv, 1997; Aviv et al., 1994) have all been documented.

Collectively, these changes will eventually result in slowness in the swallowing mechanism, a mechanism that relies on rapid, well-coordinated movements. Degeneration of nerves and sensory receptors can also result in diminished appreciation for structural position, movement, and contact.

The Preclinical State of Presbyglutition: Detectable Alterations in Swallowing

Studies comparing isolated swallows of controlled bolus size from young, healthy subjects to those of older, healthy subjects have illuminated numerous changes associated with aging. Range of motion in pharyngeal structures has been noted and attributed to the need to compensate for other changes in deglutition, such as reduced duration of upper esophageal sphincter opening (Logemann, Pauloski, Rademaker, & Kahrilas, 2002; Logemann, Pauloski, Rademaker, Colangelo, Kahrilas, & Smith, 2000). Duration of oropharyngeal movement is increased (Kendall & Leonard, 2001; Logemann et al., 2000; Rademaker, Pauloski, Colangelo, & Logemann, 1998; Robbins, Hamilton, Lof, & Kempster, 1992), as is bolus transit time (Tracy et al., 1989; Shaw et al., 1995). Decreased structural movement has also been noted (Leonard, Kendall, & McKenzie, 2004; Logemann et al., 2000). Isometric tongue pressure in older adults is significantly reduced when compared with that of younger subjects (Mortimore, Fiddes, Stephens, & Douglas, 1999; Robbins, Levine, Wood, Roecker, & Luschei, 1995), yet both groups can produce equivalent pressure during swallowing. The difference between isometric pressure and swallowing pressure is termed "reserve" pressure. With advanced age reserve diminishes, leaving a system more readily compromised by illness. Nicosia et al. (2000) also found that coincident with lower lingual isometric pressure, older adults took longer than younger adults to reach their maximal isometric pressure. Middle-aged subjects obtained higher lingual pressures with effortful swallows than did older adults (Hind, Nicosia, Roecker, Carnes, & Robbins, 2001).

Functional eating and drinking tasks bring to light differences between young adults and the elderly not found when examining isolated swallows. For example, initiation of the pharyngeal swallow begins in different areas of the mouth. In older adults, it begins with the bolus in the valleculae for masticated materials and past the ramus of the mandible for sequential liquid swallows. In young adults, however, initiation of the pharyngeal swallow begins at the anterior faucial pillars. Daniels et al. (2004) found that older adults are more likely to experience airway invasion when swallowing liquids sequentially, although they show no change in occurrence of aspiration. In a repetitive oral suction swallow test among elderly patients, subjects were noted to differ from young subjects on over 50% of the 17 parameters measured (Nilsson, Ekberg, Olsson, & Hindfelt, 1996). In single swallows, older subjects had reduced suction time and needed multiple swallows to clear the oral cavity. In forced repetitive swallowing, older subjects had reduced peak suction pressure, reduced bolus volume, longer feeding intervals, reduced swallowing capacity, polyphasic laryngeal movements, and coughing.

As mentioned earlier, not all elderly with presbyglutition will develop clinical dysphagia. Because dysphagia is not part of the normal process of aging, it is discussed in detail below in the signs of problems.

Factors Affecting Older Adults' Swallowing and Signs of Problems

Oral Health Status

Oral health issues can be present at any age, but older adults seem predisposed to these problems. Christensen (2007) cites the most common oral problems among the elderly as loss of natural teeth, xerostomia, excessive tooth wear, increased numbers of difficult-to-restore dental caries, impaired ability to perform oral hygiene, loss of alveolar bone to support removable prostheses, and periodontal disease. Gil-Montoya, Subira, Ramon, and Gonzalez-Moles (2008) found a relationship between oral health–related quality of life and risk for malnutrition in the elderly. These factors, especially with co-occurring presbyglutition, place the elderly at even greater risk for malnutrition. Xerostomia, dental issues, and taste are the factors most commonly studied in relation to swallowing and eating status in older adults. Xerostomia actually has far-reaching effects that can be seen in both dentition status and altered taste.

Chronic Dry Mouth

Mucus and saliva serve a positive and protective physiological purpose throughout the body. The respiratory, gastrointestinal, and urinogenital tracts are all lined with a mucosal surface. Mucosal tissues secrete mucus, which acts as a lubricating fluid, covering the mucosal tissue like a moving blanket. Together the mucosal tissue and its mucus covering create a layer of protection between the nonsterile external environment and the (essentially) sterile environment of the body. Mucus is an important component of saliva. The paired parotid, sublingual, and submaxillary glands as well as minor glands throughout the oral cavity produce saliva (Nagler, 2004). Three components compose saliva: the serous component that is watery, the mucus component that is more viscous, and the enzymes that initiate starch breakdown. The parotid glands contribute 25% of salivary flow, and it is all serous fluid. The sublingual glands contribute 5% of salivary flow, and it is primarily mucus. The submandibular glands contribute 70% of salivary flow, and it is a mix of serous and mucus. Salivation can be stimulated, as when eating, or unstimulated as in a rest state. The act of mastication is a known stimulant for saliva production. The constituents vary in the two states. Serous components predominate during mastication/swallowing, and mucus components predominate during an unstimulated state.

The functions of saliva are to begin the digestive process of carbohydrates; maintain a moist mouth to aid chewing, swallowing, and speaking; and act as an important participant in the immune system

(Turner & Ship, 2007). As saliva mixes with food during chewing it facilitates creation of a malleable bolus and retention of drier foods within that bolus. Oral transport of the bolus through the oral cavity and pharynx are facilitated by a moist bolus.

Chronic dry mouth can be subjective (xerostomia) as well as objective (hyposalivation; Goldie, 2007). Although it is possible to have xerostomia without hyposalivation, when it occurs in conjunction with hyposalivation, it can interfere with eating dry foods and speaking, cause discomfort in wearing dentures, and promote inflammatory conditions in the oral cavity. Xerostomia is noteworthy in patients who have undergone radiation treatment for head and neck cancer, and it is a primary characteristic of Sjögren's syndrome. Xerostomia increases with age; approximately 30% of persons aged 65 years and older experience xerostomia (Ship, Pillemer, & Baum, 2002). Many believe that the primary reason for xerostomia in older adults is as a side effect of medication (Flink, Bergdahl, Tegelberg, Rosenblad, & Lagerlof, 2008). Certain classes of drugs are well known to promote dry mouth. Anticholinergics are primary offenders. To further complicate the medication/xerostomia relationship, polypharmacy is common in the elderly, and a synergistic effect may be apparent with increasing numbers and/or classes of medications prescribed.

Dentition

The continuum of dentition seen in older adults may range from retention of a full complement of teeth to full dentures inclusive of upper and lower plates. Between these extremes are those with partial plates or missing teeth with no prosthetic. Condition of retained teeth can range from excellent to poor, and some prosthetic teeth will be well fitting, while others slip and slide. In a comparison of liquid swallows in edentulous and dentulous older adults, Yoshikawa and colleagues (2006) found that edentulous elderly exhibited greater incidence of laryngeal penetration than dentate elderly. Fucile et al. (1998) reported that older subjects with dentures tended to avoid foods that were hard or fibrous and foods with tough skins, while elderly subjects with full dentition did not avoid foods. Likewise, Shtereva (2006) concluded that those with "many" missing teeth limit food choices due to chewing problems. Nutritional deficits can ensue from such texture modifications. As mentioned earlier, the mechanical act of mastication promotes saliva production. By avoiding foods that require chewing, less saliva is produced, promoting a vicious cycle between a downgrade of texture and the presence of xerostomia.

Both dentulous and edentulous issues relate directly to xerostomia. Without a coating of mucus on the mucosa as a barrier from the hard surface of the prosthetic, dentures will lack adherence to the mucosa and move around rather than stay securely in place. Movement and the resultant rubbing of the prosthetic against tissue can cause irritation and soreness. When dentures are uncomfortable they are less likely to be worn, limiting the food textures a person will eat. For those retaining their own dentition, xerostomia can promote dental caries because the immune functions of saliva are diminished and the protective function of oral flora and fauna are disrupted. If dental caries are untreated, the bacteria associated with dental caries place someone who aspirates at greater risk for developing aspiration pneumonia (Langmore et al., 1998).

Taste

Taste appears to be essentially unchanged in aging, despite ample histological evidence that shows a change in taste buds and their related structures. This may relate to the redundancy of nerves subserving this function (Bartoshuk, 1989). Some older adults, though, do complain that food does not taste the same. Possible causes of this taste dissatisfaction are full upper dental plates covering the hard palate, impaired chewing, and altered threshold for sour taste (Yoshinaka, Yoshinaka, Ikebe, Shimanuki, & Nokubi, 2007). Medications can add a metallic taste or diminish taste (Coulter & Edwards, 1988; Elsner, 2002). Another factor is xerostomia. Saliva is necessary to maintain health and function of taste receptors. In addition, saliva is the medium in which taste substances are dissolved and then diffused to various taste receptor sites (Mese & Matsuo, 2007). A chronic bad taste in the mouth may stem from poor oral hygiene, especially in elderly adults who retain their own dentition (Langan & Yearick, 1976).

Cognitive Status

Dementia is a disease associated with aging, and cognitive impairment resulting from dementia can have deleterious effects on eating and swallowing. When discussing the phases of the swallow, the typical divisions of oral, pharyngeal, and esophageal are typically described, as in the model included earlier. There is an addition to these traditional divisions: namely, the anticipatory stage of swallowing (Leopold & Kagel, 1997). Although first described more than a decade ago, this stage of swallowing is discussed less frequently in the swallowing literature and in textbooks on the subject. The anticipatory stage recognizes cognitive, affective, motor, and sensory stimuli that precede the oral preparatory stage of swallowing. Specific examples include sensory stimuli such as smell and appearance of food, as well as pre-meal rituals such as hand washing and prayers. It also includes the hand-to-mouth aspect of eating and the modification of oral postures for accepting various utensils (e.g., cup vs. glass, fork vs. spoon). Leopold and Kagel (1997) assert that the anticipatory stage is a necessary precursor to the execution of physiologic swallowing, and that without it the cascade of oral preparation → oral transport → pharyngeal → esophageal aspects of swallowing will not transpire smoothly. The anticipatory stage of swallowing is particularly vulnerable in patients with cognitive deficits. A variety of problems eating and swallowing may be seen in patients with cognitive deficits associated with dementia. These problems will vary with type of dementia (Ikeda, Brown, Holland, Fukuhara, & Hodges, 2002; Shinagawa et al., 2009; Suh, Kim, & Na, 2009) as well as the progression of dementia. A detailed analysis is beyond the scope of this chapter. However, impaired memory may result in forgotten meals (Morley & Silver, 1988). Distractions in the environment can interfere with a patient's focus on the process of eating. Lack of recognition of food (agnosia) may result in prolonged oral phase. All of these issues can dispose patients with dementia to malnutrition, dehydration, and aspiration. Thus, monitoring during mealtime is advocated.

The Clinical State of Dysphagia

Characteristics of dysphagia are diverse, affecting all stages of the oral-pharyngeal swallow. Logemann (1998) provides a comprehensive outline of possible deficits. Oral preparatory deficits can include: reduced lip closure, tongue shaping/coordination, tongue movement, labial tension, and buccal tension resulting in food spilling anteriorly from the mouth; poor bolus control; difficulty forming a bolus; food falling into the anterior sulcus; and food falling into the lateral sulci, respectively. Oral transport deficits can include tongue thrust and delayed oral onset of swallow. Pharyngeal deficits can include delayed or absent pharyngeal swallow and reduced pharyngeal contraction, tongue base movement, velopharyngeal closure, and laryngeal elevation. As a result, a patient may aspirate before the pharyngeal swallow initiates, experience nasal regurgitation, or have food residue in the pharynx. Post-swallow residue is also a risk for aspiration.

All patients with dysphagia are at risk for aspiration, malnutrition, or dehydration. However, older adults may be more vulnerable than the young to the ramifications of these risks. If a person with dysphagia aspirates, he or she is at risk for developing aspiration pneumonia, especially when other factors, such as acid reflux and dental caries, are present (Langmore et al., 1998). Aspiration pneumonia is one of the factors associated with treatment failure in patients with community-acquired pneumonia (Genne et al., 2006; Marik & Kaplan, 2003). Those with dysphagia often have great difficulty drinking thin liquids, and water can pose the greatest problem because of its characteristic neutral taste and lack of texture. Thus, patients with dysphagia are more likely to be dehydrated. Dehydration is associated with numerous consequences such as constipation, falls, medication toxicity, urinary-tract infections, and respiratory infections (Mentes, 2006) and is associated with morbidity and mortality in older adults (Ferry, 2005). Although healthy older adults can maintain hydration as well as younger adults, older adults who are frail and/or have multiple comorbidities have difficulty maintaining hydration (Mentes, 2006). If dysphagia is added to such a scenario, then dehydration is even more likely.

Compromised nutrition from poor eating can decrease resistance to infection, exacerbate diseases, result in longer hospital stays, and increase complications and disability (Miller, Zylstra, & Standridge, 2000). In fact, nutritional risk factors, such as a 5% or greater weight loss in community-dwelling older adults, are an important predictor of institutionalization (Payette, Coulombe, Boutier, & Gray-Donald, 2000). Malnutrition and undernutrition are common yet understudied problems in the geriatric population. Few studies examine dysphagia or oral problems as potential risk factors in malnutrition in the community-dwelling elderly. As a result, little is known about the degree to which dysphagia may be a factor in malnutrition in this population. However, when dysphagia and/or oral problems *are* included in studies as potential risk factors for malnutrition, a positive association is found (Sharkey, Branch, Zohoori, Guiliani, Busby-Whitehead, & Haines, 2002; Sullivan, Martin, Flaxman, & Hagen, 1993).

Dysphagia can reduce opportunities for socialization. Persons with dysphagia may be embarrassed to eat with friends or in restaurants because of coughing or choking, which may result in increased loneliness and isolation. Over 50% of persons with known dysphagia reported that they ate less than before, and 44% had experienced weight loss in the last 12 months (Ekberg, Hamdy, Woisard, Wuttge-Hannig, & Ortega, 2002). Although 84% felt that eating should be pleasurable, only 45% found that it was so. More than a third (36%) indicated they avoided eating with others, and 41% indicated that they experienced anxiety or panic during mealtimes.

Strategies to Help Older Adults' Swallowing

Traditional testing of swallowing function can be employed to determine presence of dysphagia, including a clinical evaluation of dysphagia, modified barium swallow (MBS), or endoscopy. Supplemental testing with pulse oximetry, cervical auscultation, and other measures can also be used. These assessment techniques have been thoroughly described elsewhere (Langmore, 2001; Logemann, 1993; Murray, 1999).

It is important to recognize that dysphagia from etiologies such as stroke, traumatic head injury, or head and neck cancer in older adults may be more severe than in a younger patient with a comparable injury. Comorbidities and diminished reserve capacity are likely culprits in such situations. Diminished reserve capacity also makes older adults more vulnerable to dysphagia in situations that are not usually associated with swallowing difficulties. For example, a patient from this author's caseload (Mr. X) exemplifies this well. A gentleman in his mid-70s was diagnosed with bladder cancer. At the time of diagnosis he was in otherwise excellent health and physically active. Complications from his first surgery resulted in a second operation coupled with a lengthy hospital stay. There was no sign of neurological deficit, and yet swallowing function was impaired and an MBS revealed that he consistently and silently aspirated on all textures. In addition, pharyngeal weakness was worse on the left side compared with the right side. Two weeks later, a second MBS revealed that sensation had improved, but other aspects of swallowing dysfunction remained unchanged. He was then referred for outpatient treatment.

In general, traditional approaches to enhance swallowing safety are appropriate to use with older persons. In fact, postural compensations (head turn to the left along with chin tuck) combined with a supraglottic swallow facilitated improved swallowing function in Mr. X, and he was able to eat and drink small amounts safely. The growing interest in underlying mechanisms of strength-training exercises for dysphagia (Burkhead, Sapienza, & Rosenbek, 2007) is particularly applicable to the elderly because of documented sarcopenia in this population. Not only can exercise be of benefit via muscle strengthening in documented dysphagia, leading to an enhanced swallowing function, it can be of benefit in persons who remain in the preclinical stage of presbyglutition by helping to reestablish reserve.

A compendium of studies has demonstrated that exercise regimens can promote change in swallowing in robust older adults. Lingual resistance exercise promoted increased isometric and swallowing pressures in a group of healthy elderly adults (Robbins et al., 2005). A subgroup in this study also underwent pre- and post-exercise magnetic resonance imaging (MRI), and an increase in lingual volume was noted in each participant. In a study of the effects of the Shaker exercise, a head-raising exercise to improve dysphagia, about half of healthy, elderly participants demonstrated an increase in anterior and superior hyoid movement and upper esophageal opening (Easterling, 2008). An exercise program for healthy older adults using the expiratory muscle strength trainer (EMST) showed resulting improvement in superior and anterior movement of the hyoid bone between the mandible and the larynx, facilitating laryngeal elevation and upper esophageal sphincter opening (Kim & Sapienza, 2005). Mr. X, who was able to eat small amounts of food safely with postural changes, successfully transitioned to maintaining hydration and nutrition orally with a regular diet after completing an exercise protocol with the EMST.

It can be difficult to know when an individual might benefit from swallowing diagnostic techniques or intervention strategies. Although speech-language pathologists typically rely on inpatient screening protocols and/or physician referrals, the community-dwelling elderly may be overlooked. As the beginning of this chapter emphasized, there are no clear indicators of when someone might transition from presbyglutition to dysphagia, nor is it known when deterioration of swallowing ability moves from latent to preclinical. So what can be done to improve identification of presbyglution and dysphagia in older adults?

Knowing the right questions to ask can be key in identifying swallowing problems. Edgar (2006) recently led several focus group sessions to address swallowing issues in the elderly. The participants were between 71 and 91 years with a mean of 85 years and were without history of stroke, progressive neurological disease, or head/neck cancer. Likewise, none of them had a diagnosis of dysphagia. Participants visited their physician regularly, with appointments ranging from twice yearly to four times yearly. After indicating that they did not have "swallowing" problems, participants went on to express difficulty with choking, taking pills, and taking longer to eat, while also eliminating certain foods from their diet. In addition, one subject who described noteworthy changes of very slow eating and choking on water also expressed concern about how much worse her swallowing might become as she gets older. Yet, when queried as to whether or not she mentioned any of this to her doctor, she responded, "I never thought it was important." Another participant commented that she recently took a course in cardiopulmonary resuscitation (CPR) and has had two opportunities to use the Heimlich maneuver while in the community dining area! Fifty-four percent of the participants reported that their physician never or seldom inquired about swallowing problems during their routine visits.

At the beginning of the focus group sessions, all participants denied having swallowing problems. It was not until they were asked if they choked while eating or drinking, or had eliminated certain foods from their diet, that there was realization of what "problems swallowing" truly entailed. Many healthcare professionals likely ask more probing questions about swallowing status such as "Do you cough or choke while you eat or drink?" rather than merely asking about "swallowing." Perhaps education of physicians, nurses, occupational therapists, and physical therapists regarding how to best query older adults will facilitate improved identification of patients who might benefit from diagnosis and intervention for their swallowing problems. It would appear that in order to target swallowing problems in the community-dwelling elderly semantic barriers must be overcome, suggesting that identifying dysphagia in the community-dwelling elderly may actually be a language problem.

Quick Facts

- General Swallowing Abilities of Neurologically Intact Older Adults:
  - Experience gradual deterioration of normal swallow
    - Experience the following changes during the latent phase of presbyglutition (changes not measurable by standard testing):
      - Decreased nerve conduction velocities, reduced neurotransmitter levels, atrophy, and fibrosis of muscle
      - Increase in fat content in the tongue, which rises approximately 2.7% per decade, possibly contributing to sarcopenia (i.e., age-related loss of muscle mass and strength) of the tongue
      - Laryngeal age-related changes include: reduced motor unit firing rate, atrophy and loss of laryngeal muscle fibers, ossification of laryngeal cartilage, increased irregularity of the laryngeal cartilage articular surfaces, and reduced sensation in the pharynx and larynx; these changes eventually result in slowness in the swallowing mechanism
    - Experience the following changes in the preclinical stage of presbyglutition (changes detected by testing, such as x-ray and endoscopy):
      - Reduced duration of upper esophageal sphincter opening and increased duration of oropharyngeal movement and bolus transit time
      - Significant reduction in isometric tongue pressure compared with that of younger subjects, yet both older and younger adults can produce equivalent pressure during swallowing
      - Diminished reserve, making them more susceptible to swallowing problems
      - Initiation of the pharyngeal swallow begins with the bolus in the valleculae for masticated materials and past the ramus of the mandible for sequential liquid swallows
      - Need for increased multiple swallows to clear the oral cavity
      - In forced repetitive swallowing, reduced peak suction pressure, reduced bolus volume, longer feeding intervals, reduced swallowing capacity, polyphasic laryngeal movements, and coughing compared with younger adults

- Factors That Can Negatively Affect Older Adults' Eating and Swallowing:
  - Oral health factors:
    - Presence of chronic dry mouth can make it difficult to eat dry foods
    - Disruption in salivary flow, which can impede proper fit of dentures, promote dental caries in the dentulous, and promote inflammatory conditions in the oral cavity
    - Impaired dentition, which can result in ingestion of restricted food textures, placing an individual at risk for malnutrition
    - Reduced and/or altered taste from medications or hyposalivation, which may promote reduced food intake, placing an individual at risk for malnutrition
    - Medications, xerostomia, and poor oral hygiene, which can negatively affect taste
  - Cognitive factors:
    - Can interfere with the anticipatory phase of swallowing, possibly leading to a trickle-down effect in subsequent phases of swallowing, especially the oral and pharyngeal phases
- Signs That an Older Adult Should Be Referred to a Speech-Language Pathologist or Other Medical Professionals:
  - Overt complaints of difficulty eating, chewing, and/or swallowing
  - Complaints of dry mouth and/or difficulty or discomfort with dentures
  - Changes or restrictions in the types of food eaten, such as avoiding hard foods, fibrous foods, or foods with tough skins
  - Coughing or choking when eating foods, drinking liquids, and/or taking pills
  - Taking longer to eat
  - Oral preparatory deficits, including:
    - Reduced lip closure
    - Reduced tongue shaping/coordination, tongue movement, labial tension, buccal tension, which can result in food spilling anteriorly from the mouth
    - Poor bolus control
    - Difficulty forming a bolus
    - Food falling into the anterior sulcus
    - Food falling into the lateral sulci
  - Oral transport deficits, including:
    - Tongue thrust
    - Delayed oral onset of swallow

- Pharyngeal deficits, including:
  - Delayed or absent pharyngeal swallow
  - Reduced pharyngeal contraction, reduced tongue base movement, reduced velopharyngeal closure, reduced laryngeal elevation
- Strategies That Can Help Older Adults' Swallowing:
  - Implement the typical strategies used to facilitate safe swallow
  - Encourage older adults who are not experiencing dysphagia to use strengthening exercises that may help reestablish reserve strength:
    - Tongue-strengthening exercises have been shown to increase tongue mass
    - The Shaker exercise facilitates laryngeal elevation and upper esophageal sphincter opening
    - The expiratory muscle strength trainer (EMST) facilitates laryngeal elevation and upper esophageal sphincter opening with a benefit of enhancing the expulsive aspect of cough

Discussion Questions

1. What, if any, changes have you noticed in the eating patterns of the elderly individuals in your life? Are any of these changes concerning?
2. Older adults who experience swallowing problems often associate their difficulties with aging and fail to mention these problems to their physician. What can SLPs do to promote awareness of swallowing difficulties and dysphagia in settings such as continuing-care retirement communities or long-term care facilities?
3. Are there reasons other than the side effects of medications that make the elderly more susceptible to developing xerostomia?
4. The study by Robbins et al. (2005) had elderly participants compress an air-filled bulb between their tongue and hard palate. If you did not have such a device, what similar activities could you have older adults do in order to address lingual resistance?

References

Aviv, J. E. (1997). Effects of aging on sensitivity of the pharyngeal and supraglottic areas. *American Journal of Medicine, 103*, 74S–76S.

Aviv, J. E., Martin, J. H., Jones, M. E., Wee, T. A., Diamond, B., Keen, M. S. et al. (1994). Age-related changes in pharyngeal and supraglottic sensation. *Annals of Otology, Rhinology, and Laryngology, 103*, 749–752.

Bartoshuk, L. M. (1989). Taste: Robust across the age span? *Annals of the New York Academy of Sciences, 561*, 65–75.

Bloem, B. R., Lagaay, A. M., Van Beek, W., Haan, J., Roos, R. A. C., & Wintzen, A. R. (1990). Prevalence of subjective dysphagia in community residents aged over 87. *British Medical Journal, 300*, 721–722.

Burkhead, L. M., Sapienza, C. M., & Rosenbek, J. C. (2007). Strength-training exercise in dysphagia rehabilitation: Principles, procedures, and directions for future research. *Dysphagia, 22*, 251–265.

Casiano, R., Ruiz, P., & Goldstein, W. (1994). Histopathologic changes in the aging human cricoarytenoid joint. *Laryngoscope, 104*, 533–538.

Christensen, G. J. (2007). Providing oral care for the aging patient. *Journal of the American Dental Association, 138*, 239–242.

Coulter, D. M., & Edwards, R. (1988). Cough and angiotension converting enzyme inhibitors. *British Medical Journal, 296*, 863.

Daniels, S. K., Corey, D. M., Hadskey, L. D. et al. (2004). Mechanism of sequential swallowing during straw drinking in healthy young and older adults. *Journal of Speech, Language, and Hearing Research, 47*, 33–45.

Easterling, C. (2008). Does an exercise aimed at improving swallow function have an effect on vocal function in the healthy elderly? *Dysphagia, 23*, 317–326.

Edgar, J. (2006). *Aging swallow.* Proposal Development Award, Washington University Center for Aging.

Ekberg, O., Hamdy, S., Woisard, V., Wuttge-Hannig, A., & Ortega, P. (2002). Social and psychological burden of dysphagia: Its impact on diagnosis and treatment. *Dysphagia, 17*, 139–146.

Elsner, R. J. F. (2002). Changes in eating behavior during the aging process. *Eating Behaviors, 3*, 15–43.

Ferry, M. (2005). Strategies for ensuring good hydration in the elderly. *Nutrition Reviews, 63*, S22–S29.

Flink, H., Bergdahl, M., Tegelberg, A., Rosenblad, A., & Lagerlof, F. (2008). Prevalence of hyposalivation in relation to general health, body mass index and remaining teeth in different age groups of adults. *Community Dentistry and Oral Epidemiology, 36*, 523–531.

Fucile, S., Wright, P. M., Chan, I., Yee, S., Langlias, M., & Gisel, E. G. (1998). Functional oral-motor skills: Do they change with age? *Dysphagia, 13*, 195–201.

Genne, D., Sommer, R., Kaiser, L., Saaïdia, A., Pasche, A., Unger, P. F. et al. (2006). Analysis of factors that contribute to treatment failure in patients with community-acquired pneumonia. *European Journal of Clinical Microbiology and Infectious Disease, 25*, 159–166.

Gil-Montoya, J. A., Subira, C., Ramon, J. M., & Gonzalez-Moles, M. A. (2008). Oral health-related quality of life and nutritional status. *Journal of Public Health Dentistry, 68*, 88–93.

Goldberg, J., & Wittes, J. (1981). The evaluation of medical screening procedures. *American Statistician, 35*, 4–11.

Goldie, M. P. (2007). Xerostomia and quality of life. *International Journal of Dermatology, 5*, 60–61.

Groher, M., & Bukatman, R. (1986). The prevalence of swallowing disorders in two teaching hospitals. *Dysphagia, 1*, 3–6.

Hind, J. A., Nicosia, M. A., Roecker, E. B., Carnes, M. L., & Robbins, J. (2001). Comparison of effortful and noneffortful swallows in healthy middle-aged and older adults. *Archives of Physical Medicine and Rehabilitation, 82*, 1661–1665.

Ikeda, M., Brown, J., Holland, A. J., Fukuhara, R., & Hodges, J. R. (2002). Changes in appetite, food preference, and eating habits in frontotemporal dementia and Alzheimer's disease. *Journal of Neurology, Neurosurgery, and Psychiatry, 73*, 371–376.

Kahn, A., & Kahane, J. (1986). India ink pinprick assessment of age-related changes in the cricoarytenoid joint (CAJ) articular surfaces. *Journal of Speech, Language, and Hearing Research, 29*, 536–543.

Kendall, K., & Leonard, R. (2001). Hyoid movement during swallowing in older patients with dysphagia. *Archives of Otolaryngology—Head and Neck Surgery, 127*, 1224–1229.

Kim, J., & Sapienza, C. M. (2005). Implications of expiratory muscle strength training for rehabilitation of the elderly: Tutorial. *Journal of Rehabilitation Research and Development, 42*, 211–224.

Kuhlemeier, K. (1994). Epidemiology and dysphagia. *Dysphagia, 9*, 209–217.

Langan, M. J., & Yearick, E. S. (1976). The effects of improved oral hygiene on taste perception and nutrition of the elderly. *Journal of Gerontology, 31*, 413–418.

Langmore, S. (2001). *Endoscopic evaluation and treatment of swallowing disorders.* New York: Thieme.

Langmore, S., Terpenning, M., Schork, A., Chen, Y., Murray, J. T., Lopatin, D. et al. (1998). Predictors of aspiration pneumonia: How important is dysphagia? *Dysphagia, 13*, 69–81.

Leonard, R., Kendall, K., & McKenzie, S. (2004). Structural displacements affecting pharyngeal constriction in nondysphagic elderly and nonelderly adults. *Dysphagia, 19*, 133–141.

Leopold, N. A., & Kagel, M. C. (1997). Dysphagia—ingestion or deglutition? A proposed paradigm. *Dysphagia, 12*, 202–207.

Logemann, J. A. (1993). *Manual for the videofluorographic study of swallowing.* Austin, TX: Pro-Ed.

Logemann, J. A. (1998). *Evaluation and treatment of swallowing disorders.* Austin, TX: Pro-Ed.

Logemann, J. A., Pauloski, B. R., Rademaker, A. W., Colangelo, L. A., Kahrilas, P. J., & Smith, C. H. (2000). Temporal and biomechanical characteristics of oropharyngeal swallow in younger and older men. *Journal of Speech, Language, and Hearing Research, 43*, 1264–1274.

Logemann, J. A., Pauloski, B. R., Rademaker, A. W., & Kahrilas, P. J. (2002). Oropharyngeal swallow in younger and older women: Videofluoroscopic analysis. *Journal of Speech, Language, and Hearing Research, 45*, 434–445.

Luschei, E. S., Ramig, L. O., Baker, K. L., & Smith, M. E. (1999). Discharge characteristics of laryngeal single motor units during phonation in young and older adults and in persons with Parkinson disease. *Journal of Neurophysiology, 81*, 2131–2139.

Malmgren, L. T., Fisher, P., Jones, C., Bookman, L., & Uno, T. (2000). Numerical densities of myonuclei and satellite cells in muscle fiber types in the aging human thyroarytenoid muscle: An immunohistochemical and stereological study using confocal laser scanning microscopy. *Otolaryngology—Head and Neck Surgery, 123*, 377–384.

Marik, P. E., & Kaplan, D. (2003). Aspiration pneumonia and dysphagia in the elderly. *Chest, 124*, 328–336.

Mentes, J. (2006). Oral hydration in older adults: Greater awareness is needed in preventing, recognizing, and treating dehydration. *American Journal of Nursing, 106*, 40–49.

Mese, H., & Matsuo, R. (2007). Salivary secretion, taste and hyposalivation. *Journal of Oral Rehabilitation, 34*, 711–723.

Miller, K. E., Zylstra, R. G., & Standridge, J. B. (2000). The geriatric patient: A systematic approach to maintaining health. *American Family Physician, 61*, 1089–1104.

Monemi, M., Liu, J., Thornell, L., & Eriksson, P. (2000). Myosin heavy chain composition of the human lateral pterygoid and digastric muscles in young adults and elderly. *Journal of Muscle Research and Cell Motility*, 21, 303–312.

Morley, J. E., & Silver, A. J. (1988). Anorexia in the elderly, *Neurobiology of Aging*, 9, 9–16.

Mortimore, I. L., Fiddes, P., Stephens, S., & Douglas, N. J. (1999). Tongue protrusion force and fatigueability in male and female subjects. *European Respiratory Journal*, 14, 191–195.

Murray, J. (1999). *Manual of dysphagia assessment in adults*. San Diego, CA: Singular Publishing.

Nagler, R. M. (2004). Salivary glands and the aging process: Mechanistic aspects, health-status and medicinal-efficacy monitoring. *Biogerontology*, 5, 223–233.

Nicosia, M. A., Hind, J. A., Roecker, E. B., Carnes, M., Doyle, J., Dengel, G. A. et al. (2000). Age effects on the temporal evolution of isometric and swallowing pressure. *Journal of Gerontology: Medical Sciences*, 55A, M634–M640.

Nilsson, H., Ekberg, O., Olsson, R., & Hindfelt, B. (1996). Quantitative aspects of swallowing in an elderly nondysphagic population. *Dysphagia*, 11, 180–184.

Payette, H., Coulombe, C., Boutier, V., & Gray-Donald, K. (2000). Nutrition risk factors for institutionalization in a free-living functionally dependent elderly population. *Journal of Clinical Epidemiology*, 53, 579–587.

Rademaker, A. W., Pauloski, B. R., Colangelo, L. A., & Logemann, J. A. (1998). Age and volume effects on liquid swallowing function in normal women. *Journal of Speech, Language, and Hearing Research*, 41, 275–284.

Robbins, J., Gangnon, R. E., Theis, S. M., Kays, S. A., Hewitt A. L., & Hind, J. A. (2005). The effects of lingual exercise on swallowing in older adults. *Journal of the American Geriatrics Society*, 53, 1483–1489.

Robbins, J., Hamilton, J. W., Lof, G. L., & Kempster, G. B. (1992). Oropharyngeal swallowing in normal adults of different ages. *Gastroenterology*, 103, 823–829.

Robbins, J., Levine, R., Wood, J., Roecker, E. B., & Luschei, E. (1995). Age effects on lingual pressure generation as a risk factor for dysphagia. *Journals of Gerontology Series A: Biological Sciences and Medical Sciences*, 50, M257–262.

Rother, P., Wohlgemuth, B., Wolff, W., & Rebentrost, I. (2002). Morphometrically observable aging changes in the human tongue. *Annals of Anatomy*, 184, 159–164.

Sharkey, J., Branch, L., Zohoori, N., Guiliani, C., Busby-Whitehead, J., & Haines, P. (2002). Inadequate nutrient intakes among homebound elderly and their correlation with individual characteristics and health-related factors. *American Journal of Clinical Nutrition*, 76, 1435–1445.

Shaw, D. W., Cook, I. J., Gabb, M., Holloway, R. H., Simula, M. E., Panagopoulos, V. et al. (1995). Influence of normal aging on oral-pharyngeal and upper esophageal sphincter function during swallowing. *American Journal of Physiology Gastrointestinal and Liver Physiology*, 268, G389–396.

Shinagawa, S., Adachi, H., Toyota, Y., Mori, T., Matsumoto, I., Fukuhara, R. et al. (2009). Characteristics of eating and swallowing problems in patients who have dementia with Lewy bodies. *International Psychogeriatrics*, 21, 520–525.

Ship, J. A., Pillemer, S. R., & Baum, B. J. (2002). Xerostomia and the geriatric patient. *Journal of the American Geriatrics Society*, 50, 535–543.

Shtereva, N. (2006). Aging and oral health related to quality of life in geriatric patients. *Rejuvenation Research*, 9, 355–357.

Suh, M. K., Kim, H., & Na, D. L. (2009). Dysphagia in patients with dementia: Alzheimer versus vascular. *Alzheimer Disease and Associated Disorders*, 23, 178–184.

Sullivan, D., Martin, W., Flaxman, N., & Hagen, J. (1993). Oral health problems and involuntary weight loss in a population of frail elderly. *Journal of the American Geriatric Society, 41,* 725–731.

Takeda, N., Thomas, G. R., & Ludlow, C. L. (2000). Aging effects on motor units in the human thyroarytenoid muscle. *Laryngoscope, 110,* 1018–1025.

Tracy, J. F., Logemann, J. A., Kahrilas, P. J., Jacob, P., Kobara, M., & Krugler, C. (1989). Preliminary observations on the effects of age on oropharyngeal deglutition. *Dysphagia, 4,* 90–94.

Turner, M. D., & Ship, J. A. (2007). Dry mouth and its effects on the oral health of elderly people. *Journal of the American Dental Association, 138,* 15S–20S.

Weismer, G., & Liss, J. (1991). Speech motor control and aging. In D. Ripich (Ed.), *Handbook of geriatric communication disorders* (pp. 205–226). Austin, TX: Pro-Ed.

Yoshikawa, M., Yoshida, M., Nagasaki, T., Tanimoto, K., Tsuga, K., & Akagawa, Y. (2006). Influence of aging and denture use on liquid swallowing in healthy dentulous and edentulous older people. *Journal of the American Geriatrics Society, 54,* 444–449.

Yoshinaka, M., Yoshinaka, M. F., Ikebe, K., Shimanuki, Y., & Nokubi, T. (2007). Factors associated with taste dissatisfaction in the elderly. *Journal of Oral Rehabilitation, 34,* 497–502.

Chapter 9

Principles of the WHO *International Classification of Functioning, Disability, and Health*: Applications for the Community-Dwelling Elderly Population

Travis T. Threats, PhD, CCC-SLP

Introduction

The World Health Organization (WHO, 1945) defines health as "a state of complete physical, mental and social wellbeing and not merely the absence of disease or infirmity." In this broad definition of health, someone does not have to be "sick" in order to have a reduction in health. It eliminates an artificial dichotomy between being healthy and not being healthy, and contributes toward the current understanding of health as a continuum. For example, a person who has had a stroke is not ill in the sense that he or she needs immediate medical attention. However, that person may have reduced mental and social well-being and, thus, not be in optimum health according to WHO. Another person who has had the exact same stroke neurologically might, despite some level of impairment, be fully engaged in his or her environment and, therefore, have considerable mental and social well-being. In a medical system, the person who is not healthy may have a variety of services available to help, whereas the person deemed healthy may have no services available.

The WHO definition of health is important in discussions about the elderly population. What is considered a healthy elderly person? What makes society think a given elderly person is healthy while another is considered unhealthy? Is it possible for a 90-year-old person to truly be considered in good health? Is it possible that persons that some would consider as unhealthy would view themselves as healthy?

Despite WHO's expansion definition of health, its method of measuring health has been the traditional one of diagnosis. The most broadly used WHO classification system is the *International Statistical Classification of Diseases and Related Health Problems*, 10th revision (ICD-10; WHO, 2007), which was first developed in 1893 as the *Bertillon Classification of International List of Causes of Death* (Peterson & Rosenthal, 2005). The ICD was initially conceived as a list of diseases that could kill a person. It later expanded to disorders that did not immediately cause death, such as chronic diseases and injuries. However, its intent is still on conditions that could, left untreated, lead to death. The ICD continues to be a coding system for the diagnosis of diseases. A medical diagnosis is often the sum total of many individual symptoms, and its main purpose is to enable a physician to prescribe a given medical treatment such as prescription drugs or surgery. However, a medical diagnosis does not necessarily predict how persons function or how individuals view their condition. Thus, two people could both have what is considered moderate arthritis. One person with this disease stays mostly confined to bed and trips around the house. The other person holds a job and is involved in many civic organizations. One person who has had a stroke may have a large extended and close family that helps out whenever needed. Another person with the same extent of brain damage from a stroke lives alone with no family or close friends available. For both sets of patients described above, their ICD-coded diagnoses could not alone be used to plan effective intervention or even predict the likelihood of there being secondary diseases such as deep vein thrombosis (DVT) or depression.

There is overlap between the ICD and *International Classification of Functioning, Disability, and Health* (ICF) because both taxonomies classify impairments in various body systems. The ICD's primary purpose is to generate diagnoses of diseases, while the ICF provides information on functioning associated with various health conditions. The ICF is purely descriptive, and nothing about a given code implies a certain course of treatment; therefore, the ICF must be used holistically. Disease or impairment may be experienced very differently in two individuals, and similar functioning may occur in widely disparate health conditions. Thus, together the ICD and the ICF are intended to provide a complementary and meaningful picture of the health of people or populations.

The Need for a Functional Classification System

There has been growing recognition around the world that building a health system primarily concerning acute illness and disease does not take into account the broad issues needed to work toward having a healthy and productive society (Brundtland, 2002). With medical advances also comes increased longevity, which leads to more persons with chronic health conditions. In other times these persons would have died, but now they live. Having saved so many people's lives, the health care system must attend to the quality of their lives.

The National Committee of Vital and Health Statistics (NCVHS), an academic medical advisory board of the Department of Health and Human Services of the United States, defines functional health as the following:

> Functional status is variously defined in the health field, by clinicians with different emphases as well as in different policy contexts. This NCVHS project uses a broad view of functional status that covers both the individual carrying out activities of daily living and the individual participating in life situations and society. These two broad areas include (1) basic physical and cognitive activities such as walking or reaching, focusing attention, and communicating, as well as the routine activities of daily living, including eating, bathing, dressing, transferring, and toileting; and (2) life situations such as school or play for children and, for adults, work outside the home or maintaining a household. Functional limitations occur when a person's capacity to carry out such activities or performance of such activities is compromised due to a health condition or injury and is not compensated by environmental factors (including physical, social, and attitudinal factors). Functional status is affected by physical, developmental, behavioral, emotional, social, and environmental conditions. This conception encompasses the whole person, as engaged in his or her physical and social environment. It applies across the life span, although interpretation of functional status differs for different age groups. (NCVHS, 2001, p. 2)

This same report goes on to state the following concerning functional health status information in medical records: "The point has already been made that administrative data generally do not include information on functional status. The significance of this fact is that information on this dimension of health—increasingly the sine qua non for understanding health—is not available to the healthcare system (e.g., insurers and health plans), nor to the researchers, public health workers, and policy makers who depend on administrative data. What is needed, therefore, is a standardized code set that will enable providers, with minimal burden, to include functional status information in administrative data" (p. 6).

Development of the ICF

To capture the different levels of health and functioning, the World Health Organization published the *International Classification of Impairments, Disabilities, and Handicaps* (ICIDH) in 1980. This version was published for discussion purposes only. The goal was to provide a unified standard language for describing human functioning and disability as an important component of health, similar to how WHO's *International Statistical Classification of Diseases and Related Health Problems-10* (WHO, 2007) has set the standard for the reporting and viewing of diseases and illnesses. It was successful in garnering substantial discussion regarding aspects of disability and their relationship to health. Although useful as a general framework, the 1980 ICIDH lacked a comprehensive classification system that could be used in health systems. It was criticized internationally, especially by disability rights groups, because of its conceptual limitations (Hurst, 2003). Significant limitations were the assumptions that disabilities were primarily consequences of diseases and that there was a direct and unidirectional relationship between disease and disability. Thus, the 1980 ICIDH demonstrated a traditional medical orientation toward disability. Another objection was the use of the term *handicap*, which was viewed as reflecting an inherent trait of the person as opposed to a societal issue of the marginalization of persons with disability in society. With increasing knowledge, experience, and research regarding functioning and disability, it was evident that a significant revision was necessary.

In 1993 the WHO began this needed revision, and the finished product was published in 2001. The *International Classification of Functioning, Disability, and Health* (ICF; WHO, 2001) includes operational definitions for all categories and individual items, a complete coding system, neutral terminology, inclusion of environmental factors, and more input from socially oriented models of disability. Because the 1980 framework was frequently used worldwide, there is understandable confusion concerning the terminology and the ICF, with many erroneously believing that the same framework underlies both.

The World Health Organization considers the ICD and the ICF to be a set of classifications systems that used together can fully explain the health of individuals and populations. For example, for a given ICD diagnostic code, one can ask what are the relevant decreases in function seen with that disorder. The ICF Research Branch of the WHO Collaboration Center of the Family of International Classifications in Germany has taken the lead to develop ICF core sets based on ICD codes for a wide variety of diseases, such as rheumatoid arthritis (Stucki et al., 2004) and depression (Cieza et al., 2004). In addition, the core sets have included a combination of disease and healthcare settings such as ones on cardiopulmonary conditions in acute hospital stays (Boldt & Grill et al., 2005), and neurological patients with post-acute rehabilitation settings (Boldt & Brach et al., 2005). In addition, ICF codes can be used to describe decreases in function that cannot reliably be ascribed to a particular disease. An example would be an elderly person who exhibits difficulty with complex memory tasks, but not to the level that could be considered as dementia, and neurological imaging tests reveal no brain pathology.

The ICF has been adopted and used widely in the field of communication disorders, as well as in medicine, physical therapy, occupational therapy, recreational therapy, and nursing. The ICF was first used as the framework for the field by the American Speech-Language-Hearing Association in its Scope of Practice document in 2001. It is still included as the framework for both the Scope of Practice for Speech-Language Pathology–2007 (ASHA, 2007) and the Scope of Practice for Audiology–2004 (ASHA, 2004). Internationally, the ICF has been researched, taught, and put into clinical practice in the field of communication disorders (Threats, 2006).

The ICF was developed for the following purposes: (1) collection of statistical data concerning functioning and disability, including those used in population studies; (2) clinical research, such as the measurement of outcomes, quality of life, or impact of environmental factors on disability; (3) clinical use, such as needs assessment, matching treatments with specific conditions, program outcome evaluation, and for rehabilitation documentation; (4) social policy use, including social security planning, governmental oversight of disability programs, and policy decision making; and (5) educational use in curriculum design to raise awareness of functional health and disability issues. These five uses have been discussed in relationship to the field of communication disorders (Brown & Hasselkus, 2008; Mulhorn & Threats, 2008; Skarakis-Doyle & Doyle, 2008; Threats, 2008; Worrall & Hickson, 2008). By attempting a system that can address such diverse uses, the WHO intends not just to produce a classification system but to systematically and comprehensively reorient the healthcare system to look at issues of functioning as seriously as the system currently addresses diseases.

Description of the ICF

The ICF is based on a biopsychosocial approach that allows clinicians and researchers to document a wide range of human functioning from biological, individual, and societal perspectives. The classification system is composed of two parts: Functioning and Disability, and Contextual Factors. The Functioning and Disability part consists of the three components of Body Function, Body Structure, and Activities/Participation. The second part, Contextual Factors, consists of the two components of Environmental Factors and Personal Factors. All of the individual items of the ICF have operational definitions and examples. Each code is modified by one or more qualifiers to indicate the extent or nature of the limitation or restriction on that function. The first qualifier for all of the Body Structure, Body Function, and Activities/Participation codes is a universal qualifier that can denote five levels of severity: 0, no problem; 1, mild problem; 2, moderate problem; 3, severe problem; and 4, complete problem. Thus, a moderate difficulty with time management (b1642) would be coded as b1642.2.

The Body Structure component of the classification is defined as the "anatomic parts of the body such as organs, limbs, and their components" (WHO, 2001, p. 8). Two qualifiers are used with the individual codes. The first qualifier indicates overall severity, and the second one indicates the nature of the change to the given body structure, such as a bilateral or unilateral impairment. For example, 100.1 would indicate mild severity of vocal fold function; 100.12 would indicate that the mild severity was unilateral, as opposed to 100.11, which would indicate bilateral vocal fold dysfunction.

The Body Function component is defined as the "physiological and psychological functions of body systems" (WHO, 2001, p. 8). The eight Body Function chapters are as follows: (1) Mental functions; (2) Sensory functions and pain; (3) Voice and speech functions; (4) Functions of the cardiovascular, haematological, immunological, and respiratory systems; (5) Functions of the digestive, metabolic, and endocrine systems; (6) Genitourinary and reproductive functions; (7) Neuromusculoskeletal and movement-related functions; and (8) Functions of the skin and related structures. This component includes a wide range of functions concerning cognition, communication (language, voice, speech, fluency), and swallowing. Only the first universal qualifier is used to modify these codes. To use a previous example, a moderate difficulty with time management would be coded as b1642.2.

The Activities/Participation component of the ICF describes the functional status of persons. It consists of nine chapters that enable the user to comprehensively assess a wide variety of human behaviors, including (1) Learning and applying knowledge; (2) General tasks and demands; (3) Communication; (4) Mobility; (5) Self-care; (6) Domestic life;

(7) Interpersonal interactions and relationships; (8) Major life areas; and (9) Community, social, and civic life. Items in this component can be modified by three primary qualifiers, all of which still use the 0 through 4 severity rating system. The first qualifier, "performance," is designed to describe how a person is functioning in his or her current environment on a given life skill. The second qualifier, "capacity without assistance," describes how a person functions on a given task in a structured and standardized environment, such as in a clinic room or a research laboratory. This environment is designed to not have any overt barriers or facilitators when an individual executes the tasks. The third qualifier, "capacity with assistance," is used to code an individual's capacity in a highly facilitative environment using both assistive devices and personal assistance. In other words, can the person successfully execute the act if given sufficient cues or other assistance? This qualifier could be used as a prognostic indicator for the ability to benefit from intervention.

The Contextual Factors component includes two aspects, Environmental Factors and Personal Factors. Environmental Factors are defined as the "physical, social, and attitudinal environment in which people live and conduct their lives" (WHO, 2001, p. 16–17). It includes aspects that are external to a person's control and can have either a positive (facilitative) or negative (barrier) effect on functioning. Unlike the other components, the coding for Environmental Factors can reflect a positive or negative aspect. For example, ".+2" would indicate a moderate facilitator in the person's environment, and ".2" would indicate a moderate barrier in the person's environment. The five chapters of the Environmental Factors component are (1) Products and technology; (2) Natural environment and human-made changes to environment; (3) Support and relationships; (4) Attitudes; and (5) Services, systems, and policies.

Personal Factors are not coded in the ICF but are included in the framework because it is acknowledged that they play an important role in the disablement process. Personal factors are aspects of a person's background that are not directly part of the health condition affecting the level of functioning. These factors include age, race, gender, educational background, coping styles, past experience, upbringing, personality, social background, other health conditions, and lifestyle.

The ICF is not widely used in educational and health settings within the United States (Iezzoni, 2009). However, it has been endorsed or recommended by prominent scholarly bodies such as the Institute of Medicine (Institute of Medicine, 2007), government-convened scholarly committees (Consolidated Health Initiative, 2005; NCVHS, 2001), and most rehabilitation fields, including rehabilitation nursing, occupational therapy, physical therapy, and recreational therapy (Peterson & Rosenthal, 2005). In addition, the growing attention to chronic health difficulties and disability as a crucial component of U.S. healthcare reform may aid in the adoption of the ICF. One major Medicare interme-diary, Palmetto, a subsidiary of Blue Cross/Blue Shield, is actively promot-ing the use of the ICF framework for its member medical centers and is incorporating the ICF framework in its rehabilitation definitions (Feliciano, 2007). The World Health Organization reports that there is increasing use of the ICF in rehabilitation, home health, and disability evaluations in a number of countries, including Australia, the Netherlands, Brazil, Chile, Japan, Canada, Italy, India, and Mexico (WHO, 2009).

As a classification system, the ICF is designed to provide a frame-work for assessment. Although the ICF is not an assessment tool, the framework does direct the clinician to look at all of the components of the ICF in the assessment: Body Structure, Body Function, Activity/Participation, Environmental Factors, and Personal Factors. Ideally, the assessment report would directly address each and discuss their inter-actions. This report could simply use the framework or could use the ICF codes. Hancock (2003) found that using the framework for assess-ment and subsequent intervention helped focus the rehabilitation team around patient and family needs. Hancock also found that client, pa-tient, and family satisfaction and understanding of the therapeutic process improved after the implementation of the ICF framework.

The ICF could also help organize information in patients' medical records. At present, the core medical record includes only a list of pre-vious or current diseases or disorders. Use of the ICF would elevate personal factors and environmental factors to the key components of the history. Currently, this type of information might be located in the so-cial worker's notes or other parts of the medical chart. However, this information might be crucial for successful management of patients' overall health and functioning.

Since the ICF is a broad summary measure of outcomes, it is not well suited for daily reporting of goals, such as SOAP notes. Some ICF codes for communication are quite broad, such as d335, "Producing nonverbal messages," and would not be appropriate for goals, as in "Patient will improve on ICF code d335 to 80% accuracy." Instead, the ICF could be used to measure progress every month or at the be-ginning and planned cessation of intervention. Although specific codes may not be used in daily sessions, the language of the ICF could be used in daily notes, as in "Patient reported to clinician that more comfort-able talking with friends on the phone, indicating an increase in participation in life" or "Wife of patient stated that she has learned to be a better facilitator of her husband in maintaining a conversation."

The ability of the ICF to improve healthcare data in electronic medical records has been strongly endorsed by the Consolidated Health Initiative (2005). This group has worked to develop a recommendation to the U.S. federal government of what are the essential languages and classification systems to use for an ideal U.S. universal and reciprocal electronic medical records system. Mulhorn and Threats (2008) report that improved reporting of communication disorders in medical and government epidemiologic records would increase awareness of communication disorders as a significant functional health concern.

ICF Use for Persons With Communication and Swallowing Disorders

Although the purpose of this chapter and book is to look at healthy aging adults, it is useful to discuss the literature concerning the use of the ICF to describe those communication disorders that are more likely to occur later in life. Recent articles have discussed the application of the ICF to persons with the following communication disorders: aphasia (Simmons-Mackie & Kagan, 2007), dysarthria (Dykstra, Hakel, & Adams, 2007), dementia (Hopper, 2007), dysphagia (Threats, 2007), traumatic brain injury (Larkins, 2007), hearing impairment (Hickson & Scarinci, 2007), voice disorders (Ma, Yiu, & Verdolini Abbott, 2007), and communication difficulties after a total laryngectomy (Eadie, 2007). The different components of the ICF, including Body Function, Activities and Participation, and Contextual Factors, have also been discussed concerning communication disorders (Howe, 2008; McCormack & Worrall, 2008; O'Halloran & Larkins, 2008).

A majority of individuals with neurogenic communication disorders that are acquired later in life will be community dwelling. According to classic medical thinking, these persons will not be considered ill. For example, persons do not come to the physician to check up on their aphasia every six months. The physician would instead see them to determine if they have any symptoms of a new stroke, or to monitor risk factors for another stroke. In fact, barring an acute episode, they may not have any physician visits. However, according to the ICF definition of health, these persons with a communication disability may not be in full health.

An important consideration concerning those persons with diagnosed medically based communication disorders is the possibility of other "normal" decreases in function they may manifest. For example, a patient may have dysphagia secondary to laryngeal cancer surgery. Other than a possible voice problem, this patient may not be considered to have, or even be at any risk for, a communication disorder. However, in the course of managing his postsurgical complications and dysphagia, it might be noted that the patient is not fully compliant. It may be that the written instructions were difficult for him to read secondary to visual limitations, or the instructions were given in a room with significant ambient noise. In this case, an understanding of the functional limitations associated with aging is essential to successful evaluation and intervention for persons with identified communication disorders. In the ICF framework, these functional limitations do not have to be linked to a particular disease. The ICF is simply a description and not a diagnosis, as would be captured in an ICD code.

It is also possible that a given communication disorder may be perceived as more severe because of co-occurring normal changes associated with aging. For example, a nursing home resident with moderate dementia and an accompanying hearing loss may demonstrate decreased socialization with fellow residents. The nursing home staff could interpret the increasing isolation from the group as indicative of the resident's deteriorating cognitive abilities, although at least some of the change in behavior could be due to the hearing loss. As with the previous example, there is a mix here of a traditional medical problem represented by an ICD code (dementia) along with the WHO's ICF expansion of decreased health being a reduction in some aspect of functioning (hearing loss/speech discrimination decrement).

When the Sum Equals More Than the Parts

Another complex issue concerning medical health, functional health, and aging is, at what point do you state that a person is "unhealthy?" It is clear that a person who has chronic disabling heart and lung problems and, consequently, cannot walk more than 25 yards without being out of breath is not healthy. It is equally clear that the 70-year-old who runs a marathon while also serving as a president of a successful company and who has a strong and loving family system is quite healthy.

Now consider a person who has mild arthritis, moderate visual problems, moderate hearing difficulties, mild bladder control difficulties, and mild difficulties with memory and concentration. Although not destitute, he is having some trouble paying his bills and his wife is in a depression over the recent loss of her lifelong best friend. In addition, he has begun to regret past decisions he has made in life, which worries him greatly. In a traditional view of health, this person is experiencing no more difficulty than many elderly persons might have and, therefore, would be considered in relatively good health. However, in functional health terms used by the ICF, a different picture may emerge. It is possible that a combination of his health conditions and life circumstances could significantly affect his functional health. If this person was the head of his local Knights of Columbus chapter and this affiliation was central to his identity and livelihood, then this combination could prevent him from exercising his duties or even being active in the group. If this person is self-employed, these circumstances could also affect his ability to function effectively and threaten his financial viability.

Thus, a person is a sum of his total limitations and restrictions, including Personal and Environmental factors. All of these could have an effect on one's functional health as "health" is defined by the World Health Organization. Those traits that may not seem that severe separately could add up to more than could be easily predicted. When there are disruptions in persons' overall cognitive and affective states, there are likely to be effects on communication. These could include whom they communicate with, how they communicate with others, as well as how others communicate with them. By having a more holistic view of a person's total functioning instead of just focusing on the parts, a better understanding of both the overall health and communicative health of older persons can be appreciated.

ICF and Issues in Normal Aging

One of the purposes of the ICF is to provide an alternative to having to "pathogize" any given difficulty. In traditional medical model thinking, until something reaches a critical stage of being considered a disease, it is often not provided with any intervention or services. A 90-year-old person has most likely experienced significant loss of personal relationships, such as a family member or close friends. It is a normal reaction to be despondent over these deaths, but unless the person is classified as having a clinical depression, he or she may not exist in the current medical system. Even if that individual went to see a physician, the physician might declare him or her "disease free" if no classic signs of depression are present, such as thoughts of suicide or feelings of worthlessness. This person would have failed to reach that critical threshold to be considered ill. However, with the ICF, the person might rate as having a functional health limitation on several fronts, such as on codes involving socializing with others, sense of social support, or involvement in community activities. The individual may have a variety of limitations or restrictions on life functions that may need attention but perhaps not medical intervention like taking antidepression medication.

Although the ICF categories do not represent disease symptoms, they may indicate either a developing medical problem or a life situation that could have negative medical effects. In the example above, the older person is upset about the death of significant others in life but does not exhibit the necessary symptoms to be considered in a clinical depression. The current system, at least in the United States, is often to wait until the individual is in a clinical depression and then provide intervention. Would it not be more beneficial to provide intervention before it reaches this traditional medical state? Functional health limitations often precede what are traditionally considered medical issues (Scott, Macera, Corman, & Sharpe, 1997). The decrease in community involvement can lead not only to depression but also to less vigilance in taking medications. Not taking one's medicines can result in the exacerbation of medical conditions, which, in turn, further restrict life functions and activities. As stated in the NCVHS report quoted earlier in this chapter, these life functions are increasingly recognized as legitimate health problems. Not surprisingly, those interested in public health are seeing these issues as necessary to address in order to have a healthy population.

Contextual Factors With Aging

The ICF Contextual Factors of Environmental Factors and Personal Factors are important ones to address in any discussion of normal aging. These two factors often influence each other, and it can be difficult to state which one has the most influence. From childhood to adulthood to older age, these two factors may undergo significant changes, which affects life functioning.

Environmental Factors

In the course of any person's lifetime, there are a variety of changes in one's circumstances or environment. In the beginning, one is dependent on others. Later, one may be relatively independent, such as during young unmarried adulthood. Many persons then enter a period where others depend upon them, such as a spouse or children. In later life, one may return to relative independence, as is the case with having grown children and a deceased spouse. However, in later life, one might also return to some level of dependence upon others. For example, driving might become difficult because of glaucoma, and except for familiar places, one might need for a grown child or friend to drive him or her places, or a person might start using public transportation.

How a person responds to changes in his or her life circumstances depends upon a number of factors. One factor relates to the other corresponding changes in the Environmental Factor domains. In middle age, one might be fairly financially secure. In older age, however, one may see those financial resources shrink due to age-related circumstances, such as paying for the nursing home for a spouse. As a result, the transition is not only one of aging but a shift in financial resources, which obviously can significantly affect one's life functioning. In the case of reduced financial means, it might mean not being able to belong to a country club that has been important to one's social life or having to move out of a neighborhood or even region of the country he or she has lived in for decades.

Other Environmental Factors that may demonstrate change in older age are support and relationships, healthcare services available, and attitudes of others. In support and relationships, as previously discussed, the loss of long-term relationships can be significantly disruptive to life functioning. This loss does not have to involve death. For example, after retiring, some persons "grieve" for the loss of their fellowship with other employees at a job, especially one that has been held for years.

Access to available or needed services can also be affected for older adults. As companies seek to contain costs, medical benefits such as prescription services can be limited. With increasing numbers of physicians not taking Medicare, some elders may find they can no longer see their own physicians unless they can afford to pay privately. In terms of dealing with government agencies, many older adults may have had limited experience with this particularly challenging system. This can make it difficult for them to negotiate through, or even being aware of, what government services are available. As a result, they may not be able to fully exploit the resources available to them.

Attitudes of persons who are elderly must also be given serious consideration on its possible negative effects on life functioning. The concerned attitudes are self-stereotypes and the stereotypes of others. In self-stereotypes, the person limits themselves based on stereotypical thinking. At first, this seems impossible in that stereotypes are typically thought of as attitudes toward others, not oneself. But as Gallois and Pittam (2002) have pointed out in discussion of persons' later life onset disability, some minority groups you are not born into but become later in life. Gallois and Pittam (2002) discuss persons having a stroke who are suddenly for the first time a member of a minority and disadvantaged group: "the disabled." How they respond to this new situation may be influenced by their view of persons with disabilities before they had a disability themselves. If that view was negative, they may be inclined to now have a negative view of themselves. In aging, the person may have had stereotypes about older persons and now they find themselves in that position. How will that affect their views toward their own functioning? Will they seek out treatment at the first signs of possible functional limitations, or will they assume that cognitive and mental declines are an inevitable consequence of old age? Will they seek out a hearing evaluation and accept hearing aids? It is possible that future generations of older persons may be different than the current group. Some have suggested that the baby boomers expect to have more active later years than previous older persons (Center of Health Communication, Harvard School of Public Health, 2004). However, it is yet to be seen if this group of high-expectation elders will be able to accept and adapt to some of the natural limitations that come with older age, or if their approach toward aging is to simply ignore its existence or "overcome" it.

Societal attitudes toward aging have been the subject of much research. A popular phrase when someone forgets something or makes a mistake is that one is having a "senior moment." The U.S. Federal Trade Commission had to issue a warning to a manufacturer of a product named "Senior Moment" that claimed it improved memory (Federal Trade Commission, 2004). It is interesting to note that one of the highest compliments given to an older person is that they are "80 years young," which implies that it is alright to be 80 if you do not seem to actually be 80 years old. In other words, chronologically 80 years old, but in mindset and vigor still a young person. Thus, to be 80 years old and climbing a mountain (something many 40-year-old persons cannot do) lifts the stigma of being "old." The proliferation of "anti-aging" remedies indicates that many Western cultures consider aging a disease process that can be "cured" via biochemistry or, more recently, through genetic therapies. In ICF terms, any negative societal attitudes toward elderly persons constitutes a possible Environmental Factor barrier that may restrict or limit life functioning and participation. When persons have acquired communication disorders, these negative attitudes can be as much a barrier to life participation as the actual disorder itself. Thus, such attitudes require serious consideration for the communication disorder professional.

Personal Factors

"Master status" is a sociological term that refers to the idea that knowing one attribute of a person will explain all other traits or characteristics (Marshall, 1998). It is a common component of stereotypes concerning race, religiosity, socioeconomic level, country of origin, or occupation. One of the reasons that the ICF includes Personal Factors in the framework is to recognize that any type of functional limitation or disability is just one aspect of persons' entire selves. Thus, a person who has limited mobility and is in a wheelchair could be intelligent or not, kind or not, or even tolerant of others' limitations or not. Similarly in studying the elderly population, as much as the topic is discussed and researched, there is no "elderly personality" or even a highly predictable "elderly cognitive profile" (Valdois, Joanette, Poissant, Ska, & Dehaut, 1990).

Persons' transition into older age depends upon many of the Personal Factors, including coping skills, lifestyle, personality, upbringing, education, and a number of other factors. In fact, how persons transition and thrive in older age has much to do with how they lived their lives when they were younger (Britton, Shipley, Singh-Manoux, & Marmot, 2008). Did they spend every dime as quickly as they earned it, or did they have a sustained disciplined savings plan for later years? Did they take care of their health even without any known health conditions, or did they live in an "eat, drink, and be merry, for tomorrow we may die" fashion?

Personal Factors also influence how one will respond to normal changes with aging (Steptoe, Wright, Kunz-Ebrecht, & Llifee, 2006; Yuen, Gibson, Yau, & Mitcham, 2007). Studies have looked at demographic factors such as race and socioeconomic status as indicators of how individuals approach aging. However, there are more differences than just the demographic changes often focused on in research. All persons are unique combinations of their genetics, environment, and idiosyncrasies. Some of these differences will be how they communicate with others and whom and how many people they communicate with in a typical day. Vogel and Awh (2008) have argued for looking at these differences in functioning. Using visual working memory as an example, they state:

> However, in the context of most standardized cognitive neuro-science studies, this variability across individuals is typically treated as a nuisance or as error variance, potentially obscuring differences between levels of their independent variables. Treating individual differences in this way makes sense for cognitive sciences attempting to understand how cognitive constructs such as perception, attention, and memory operate at the general level. Most cognitive neuroscientists are interested how everyone thinks, not trying to catalog and characterize the entire range of abilities across the population or understand how and why a given individual thinks differently from another. We argue that these are not mutually exclusive goals, and that by characterizing individual differences in ability within the context of sound experimental design, one can often learn a great deal more about how a cognitive process operates at a basic level. (Vogel and Awh, 2008, p. 171)

Similarly, when looking at communication disorders and their relationship with normal aging processes, both clinicians and researchers should be exploring the person in front of them, not simply the theoretical typical person. There may be additional information to learn from this combination of looking at individual differences within an experimental framework.

Interaction of Body Function Impairments With Environmental and Personal Factors

In looking at communication issues in normal aging, there is also an interaction of normal processes of aging and Environmental and Personal Factors. People are not simply pawns in their environment; they can often influence their environment. Consider the example of Bill, who withdraws from others because of a hearing decrement that makes it hard to understand others in crowds. He begins to turn down invitations to parties. Soon others start not inviting Bill to social get-togethers.

He then decides that his friends have turned against him and writes them off. He may even become depressed over the loss of friends, resulting in Bill not taking care of his personal health.

Now it is time to change some of the Contextual Factors in this story. In this case, Bill's friends realize something is amiss. One even says that Bill did not seem to hear him when he asked a question. One of the friends is a successful hearing-aid user and agrees to talk with Bill individually at his home. He convinces Bill to get his hearing tested. Bill gets fitted for a hearing aid and even takes some aural rehabilitation sessions. He fully rejoins his group and life is good for him.

The next proposed change is in Bill himself. Bill is one that accepts that some things change over time. He also reflects on other challenges in his life and that when he asked for help, he was able to overcome these difficulties. Maybe he still does not want a hearing aid but simply tells others that they will have to be in front of him and look at him when talking in a crowd. Bill could also tell people that if they want to have a full conversation with him that they have to go off to a more quiet room. Again, Bill stays in his group and life continues to stay good for him.

In the above scenarios, Bill has the same physiological change in his Body Function. However, as can be seen, the various Environmental Factors and Personal Factors influenced the ultimate outcome. In reality, the combinations and interactions of the different aspects of functioning for a given person are even more complex than the above given example.

If elderly persons need our assistance, speech-language pathologists need to meet these persons where they are. This is a broader view of diversity than is often talked about in the field. For as large as the inter-group diversity differences may be, there may be more intra-group differences. People do not start off life with the same brains, personalities, and life circumstances. Thus, it would be illogical to think that they are the same in their later years. In addition, those brains, personalities, and life circumstances might change over time in ways that would produce situations and behaviors that a person could not predict concerning their own future. These changes could be either good or negative. For some, aging is the culmination of a life's work, such as Benjamin Franklin signing the Declaration of Independence at age 80. Others are able to do something in older age that was denied to them in youth. An elderly woman who always did only what her husband told her to do may find herself as a widow being heavily involved in a political campaign and having a new circle of conversational partners and topics. Then there is the story of Alferd Williams. He was born into a sharecropper family in Arkansas when African Americans were not required to go to school. To help support his family, he worked in the cotton fields instead of ever going to school. In 1998, he ended up broke and in a homeless shelter for several weeks. But then in 2005, at age 70, he found a willing teacher and learned to read, and an entire world of communication became available to him (Dennis, 2008).

Conclusion

In conclusion, the determination of the "health" of elderly persons is multifaceted. Both functional health status and traditional indices of illness or disease must both be considered. The World Health Organization's *International Classification of Functioning, Disability, and Health* (ICF) can be used to classify functional health status at several different levels, including body functions and activities and participation. In addition, the ICF addresses aspects of persons' environments (e.g., social support and attitudes), demographics (e.g., race, gender), and personality characteristics. Health conditions and functional health status interact with environmental and personal factors to influence the quality of life for elderly persons. Increasingly, governments, healthcare systems, and healthcare providers are realizing that all aspects of health must be addressed to insure an optimum life for elderly individuals. In addition, it is being recognized that the elderly have great variability in both functional health and traditional health measures, and their reactions to these aspects of health vary widely. Although aging is unfortunately often associated only with decline, elderly persons can not only demonstrate resilience in the face of health difficulties, but also continue to grow and experience new aspects of functional health.

Quick Facts

- The World Health Organization (WHO) views health as including not just physical health but also mental and social well-being
- Functional health is increasingly being recognized by health policy and service professionals as essential in order to have a truly healthy population
- The WHO developed the *International Classification of Functioning, Disability, and Health* (ICF) to help address the important area of functional health
- The ICF framework includes Body Structures, Body Function, Activity/Participation, Environmental Factors, and Personal Factors
- The ICF framework helps elucidate the complex interactions between health, disability, and aging

- Self-perceptions and attitudes of others concerning aging can have an effect on life functioning for elderly persons
- There is wide variability in the health of elderly persons and in their approaches toward the aging process

Discussion Questions

1. Why is it helpful that the ICF provides a description and not a specific diagnosis?
2. What types of attitudes do you believe your parents and your grandparents have toward aging? Do these differ from what your attitude is toward aging?
3. Can you think of personal examples in which a medical diagnosis did not fully describe how an older person was able to function in his or her daily life?
4. How could you include principles of the ICF when evaluating an elderly adult?

References

American Speech-Language-Hearing Association. (2004). *Scope of Practice in Audiology* [Scope of Practice]. Retrieved July 12, 2009, from http://www.asha.org/policy

American Speech-Language-Hearing Association. (2007). *Scope of Practice in Speech-Language Pathology* [Scope of Practice]. Retrieved July 12, 2009, from http://www.asha.org/policy

Boldt, C., Brach, M., Grill, E., Berthou, A., Meister, K, Scheuringer, M. et al. (2005). The ICF categories identified in nursing interventions administered to neurological patients with post-acute rehabilitation needs. *Disability and Rehabilitation, 27,* 431–436.

Boldt, C., Grill, E., Wildner, M., Portenier, L., Wilke, S., Stucki, G. et al. (2005). ICF Core Set for patients with neurological conditions in the acute hospital. *Disability and Rehabilitation, 27,* 375–380.

Britton, A., Shipley, M., Singh-Manoux, A., & Marmot, M. (2008). Successful aging: The contribution of early-life and midlife risk factors. *Journal of the American Geriatrics Society, 56,* 1098–1105.

Brown, J., & Hasselkus, A. (2008). Professional associations' roles in advancing the ICF in speech-language pathology. *International Journal of Speech-Language Pathology, 10,* 78–82.

Brundtland, G. Opening address. WHO Conference on Health and Disability. Trieste, Italy, 2002. Retrieved June 24, 2008, from http://www.who.int/director-general/speeches/2002/english/20020418_disabilitytrieste.html

Center for Health Communication, Harvard School of Public Health. (2004). *Reinventing aging: Baby boomers and civic engagement.* Boston: Harvard School of Public Health.

Cieza, A., Chatterji, S., Andersen, C., Cantista, P., Herceg, M., Melvin, J. et al. (2004). ICF Core Sets for depression. *Journal of Rehabilitation Medicine, 36,* 128–134.

Consolidated Health Initiative (2005). *Consolidated Health Informatics Initiative: Standards Adoption Recommendation—Functioning and Disability.* Retrieved October 8, 2009, from http://www.ncvhs.hhs.gov/061128lt.pdf

Dennis, A. (2008). A first grader at age 70. *People, 69*, 92–99.

Dykstra, A. D., Hakel, M. E., & Adams, S. G. (2007). Application of the ICF in reduced speech intelligibility in dysarthria. *Seminars in Speech and Language, 28*, 301–311.

Eadie, T. (2007). Application of the ICF in communication after total laryngectomy. *Seminars in Speech and Language, 28*, 291–300.

Federal Trade Commission. (2004, July 13). News release: *"Senior Moment" maker neglects to prove its claims*. Accessed on June 12, 2008, from http://www.ftc.gov/opa/2004/07/nutramax.shtm

Feliciano, H. (2007). *Promoting appropriate access to care*. Presentation at ICDR State-of-the-Art Conference: New Federal Applications of the ICF. Washington, DC.

Gallois, C., & Pittam, J. (2002). *Living with aphasia: The impact and communication of self-stereotypes and other stereotypes*. Seminar presented at the 10th International Aphasia Rehabilitation Conference, Brisbane, Australia.

Hancock, H. (2003). Rehabilitation for enhanced life participation: A living well program. *Speech Pathology Online*. Retrieved October18, 2007, from http://www.speechpathology.com/articles/article_detail.asp?article_id=21

Hickson, L., & Scarinci, N. (2007). Older adults with acquired hearing impairment: Applying the ICF in rehabilitation. *Seminars in Speech and Language, 28*, 283–290.

Hopper, T. (2007). The ICF and dementia. *Seminars in Speech and Language, 28*, 273–282.

Howe, T. (2008). The ICF Contextual Factors related to speech-language pathology. *International Journal of Speech-Language Pathology, 10*, 27–37.

Hurst, R. (2003). The international disability rights movement and the ICF. *Disability and Rehabilitation, 25*, 572–576.

Iezzoni, L. (2009, June). *Are the stars aligning for the ICF in the United States?* Presentation given at the Institute for Health Policy, Massachusetts General Hospital, Harvard Medical School. Retrieved October 8, 2009, from http://www.ncvhs.hhs.gov/090610p1.pdf

Institute of Medicine. (2007). *Future of disability in America*. Washington, DC: National Academies Press.

Larkins, B. (2007). The application of the ICF in cognitive communication disorders following traumatic brain injuries. *Seminars in Speech and Language, 28*, 334–342.

Ma, E., Yiu, E., & Verdolini Abbott, K. (2007). Application of the ICF in voice disorders. *Seminars in Speech and Language, 28*, 343–350.

Marshall, G. (Ed.). (1998). *A dictionary of sociology*. Oxford: Oxford University Press.

McCormack, J., & Worrall, L. (2008). The ICF Body Functions and Structures related to speech-language pathology. *International Journal of Speech-Language Pathology, 10*, 9–17.

Mulhorn, K., & Threats, T. (2008). Speech, hearing, and communication across five national disability surveys: Results of a DISTAB study using the ICF to compare prevalence patterns. *International Journal of Speech-Language Pathology, 10*, 61–71.

National Committee on Vital and Health Statistics. (2001). *Classifying and reporting functional health status*. Washington, DC: Department of Health and Human Services.

O'Halloran, R., & Larkins, B. (2008). The ICF Activities and Participation related to speech-language pathology. *International Journal of Speech-Language Pathology, 10*, 18–26.

Peterson, D., & Rosenthal, D. (2005). The International Classification of Functioning, Disability and Health (ICF): A primer for rehabilitation educators. *Rehabilitation Education, 19*, 81–94.

Scott, W., Macera, C., Corman, C., & Sharpe, P. (1997). Functional health status as a predictor of mortality in men and women over 65. *Journal of Clinical Epidemiology, 50*, 291–296.

Simmons-Mackie, N., & Kagan, A. (2007). Application of the ICF in aphasia. *Seminars in Speech and Language, 28*, 244–253.

Skarakis-Doyle, E. & Doyle, P. (2008). The ICF as a framework for interdisciplinary doctoral education in rehabilitation: Implications for speech-language pathology. *International Journal of Speech-Language Pathology, 10*, 83–91.

Steptoe, A., Wright, C., Kunz-Ebrecht, S., & Llifee, S. (2006). Dispositional optimism and health behaviour in community-dwelling older people: Associations with healthy ageing. *British Journal of Health Psychology, 11*, 71–84.

Stucki, G., Cieza, A., Geyh, S., Battistella, L., Lloyd, J., Symmons, D. et al. (2004). ICF Core Sets for rheumatoid arthritis. *Journal of Rehabilitation Medicine, 36*, 87–93.

Threats, T. (2006). Towards an international framework for communication disorders: Use of the ICF. *Journal of Communication Disorders, 39*, 251–265.

Threats, T. (2007). Use of the ICF in dysphagia management. *Seminars in Speech and Language, 28*, 323–333.

Threats, T. (2008). Use of the ICF for clinical practice in speech-language pathology. *International Journal of Speech-Language Pathology, 10*, 50–60.

Valdois, S., Joanette, Y., Poissant, A., Ska, B., & Dehaut, F. (1990). Heterogeneity in the cognitive profile of normal elderly. *Journal of Clinical and Experimental Neuropsychology, 12*, 587–596.

Vogel, E., & Awh, E. (2008). How to exploit diversity for scientific gain: Using individual differences to constrain cognitive theory. *Current Directions in Psychological Science, 17*, 171–176.

World Health Organization. (1945). *World Health Organization Constitution.* Geneva, Switzerland. Retrieved October 18, 2007, from http://www.searo.who.int/EN/Section898/Section1441.htm

World Health Organization. (2001). *International Classification of Functioning, Disability, and Health* (ICF). Geneva, Switzerland: World Health Organization.

World Health Organization. (2007). *International Statistical Classification of Diseases and Related Health Problems–10.* Geneva, Switzerland: World Health Organization.

World Health Organization. (2009). *ICF application areas.* Retrieved October 8, 2009, from http://www.who.int/classifications/icf/appareas/en/index.html

Worrall, L., & Hickson, L. (2008). The use of the ICF in speech-language pathology research: Towards a research agenda. *International Journal of Speech-Language Pathology, 10*, 72–77.

Yuen, H., Gibson, R., Yau, M., & Mitcham, M. (2007). Actions and personal attributes of community-dwelling older adults to maintain independence. *Physical and Occupational Therapy in Geriatrics, 25*, 35–53.

Appendix

Tests for Adults

Test	Evaluates	Pros	Cons
Aphasia Diagnostic Profiles (ADP; Helm-Estabrooks, 1992)	Expression, comprehension, aphasia severity, alternative communication (e.g., gestures).	Series of brief tasks that survey a variety of abilities.	Directions are not always clear for client or clinician during testing or scoring. Does not always place person into a reliable category.
Aphasia Language Performance Scales (ALPS; Keenan & Brassell, 1975)	Reading, writing, listening, talking.	Can be given in approximately 30 minutes.	Limited items covering differing levels of difficulty for each subtest. Clients need adequate auditory comprehension in order to complete the reading section.
Apraxia Battery for Adults, 2nd edition (ABA-2; Dabul, 2003)	Diadochokinetic rate, increasing word length, limb apraxia, oral apraxia, latency time and utterance time for polysyllabic words.	Directions for clients are easy to follow.	Administration time may be increased for more severe impairments.
Arizona Battery for Communication Disorders of Dementia (ABCD; Bayles & Tomoeda, 1993)	Mental status, immediate and delayed story retelling, following commands, naming and repetition, word learning, reading comprehension, and figure copying. Includes screening tasks for speech discrimination and visual perception.	Includes normative data for older and younger healthy adults. Normative data also for persons with dementia resulting from Alzheimer's disease and Parkinson's disease.	Is not suitable for individuals with severe dementia.

Assessment of Intelligibility of Dysarthric Speech (AIDS; Yorkston & Beukelman, 1984)	Intelligibility and speaking rate of persons with dysarthria using phonetically balanced items.	Allows for measures of intelligibility in single words and sentences. Provides norms for speaking rate.	Clinician needs another person to listen to and transcribe client responses. Speaking rate norms are not specific to older adults.
Bilingual Verbal Ability Tests (BVAT; Munoz-Sandoval, Cummins, Alvarado, & Ruef, 2005)	Naming pictures.	Tests knowledge of bilinguals using a combination of two languages, including but not limited to English, Arabic, Chinese, French, German, Hindi, Italian, Russian, Spanish, and Turkish.	Best administered by a bilingual examiner.
Boston Assessment of Severe Aphasia (BASA; Helm-Estabrooks, Ramsberger, Morgan, & Nicholas, 1989)	Social greetings, simple conversation, yes/no questions, orientation, bucco-facial praxis, sustained "ah," singing, repetition, limb praxis, comprehension of number symbols, naming of objects and famous faces, reading, signing name.	Designed specifically for persons with severe aphasia. Comprehensive in nature and provides good baseline data for multiple modalities.	Can be awkward to administer at bedside because of all the cards and objects the clinician needs.
Boston Diagnostic Aphasia Examination, 3rd edition (BDAE-3; Goodglass, Kaplan, & Barresi, 2001)	Conversational and expository speech, auditory comprehension, oral expression, understanding written language, writing.	Is comprehensive and provides good baseline data for multiple modalities. Classifies patients into type of aphasia.	Administration time may be long (1 to 3 hours). Not well-suited for individuals with severe aphasia.

(continues)

Tests for Adults *(Continued)*

Test	Evaluates	Pros	Cons
Boston Naming Test, 2nd edition (BNT-2; Kaplan, Goodglass, & Weintraub, 2001)	The ability to name 60 line drawings of objects that vary in familiarity (e.g., bench, abacus).	Used with various age groups (ages 6 through adulthood). Straightforward to use. Has been translated into many languages.	Clients may not have known target item premorbidly.
Cognitive Linguistic Quick Test (CLQT; Helm-Estabrooks, 2001)	Attention, memory, language, executive function, visuospatial skills.	Can generally be given in 15 to 30 minutes. Includes verbal and nonverbal tasks. Has an English and Spanish version.	Older adults could have age-related vision declines that would result in poor performance on visuospatial tasks, but which may not truly reflect their cognitive abilities.
Communication Activities of Daily Living, 2nd edition (CADL-2; Holland, Frattali, & Fromm, 1999)	Reading, writing, using numbers, social interactions, contextual and nonverbal communication, explaining humor and absurdities.	Assesses communication in situations that resemble daily living.	Need to have a telephone and someone to call.
Dworkin-Culatta Oral Mechanism Examination and Treatment System (Dworkin & Culatta, 1980)	Oral and speech apraxia.	Is generally easy to score. Can be used with young children and adults.	Can take 1 to 2 hours to administer. Not standardized.
Functional Communication Profile-Revised (FCP; Kleiman, 2003)	Sensory skills (e.g., hearing, vision), motor abilities (e.g., grasp, head and trunk positioning), behavior, attentiveness, receptive language, expressive language, pragmatic/social abilities, speech, voice, oral, fluency, nonverbal communication.	Includes observation of clients by clinician. Assesses communication in situations that resemble daily living.	No normative data. Clinicians need to provide their own materials for testing.

Independent Living Scales (Loeb, 1996)	Orientation, competence in activities of daily living, such as managing money, managing home and transportation (e.g., how to regulate temperature of home, how to find out cost of bus fare), health and safety (e.g., how to call police, how to know when it is safe to cross the street), and mental health of the patient.	Functional test that relates to independent daily living.	Patients may not do well if they cannot express themselves verbally.
Mann Assessment of Swallowing Ability (MASA; Mann, 2002)	Likelihood for presence of dysphagia and aspiration and the severity of impairment.	Can be used to help make dietary recommendations. Measures other pertinent information such as attention, cooperation, and auditory comprehension.	Normative data is specific to persons who have suffered strokes.
Mini Inventory of Right Brain Injury, 2nd edition (MIRBI-2; Pimental & Kingsbury, 2000)	Letter identification, reading, writing, subtraction, clock drawing, presence of left-side neglect, understanding emotional, humorous, and figurative language.	Can generally be administered in 30 minutes. One of the few tests that is specifically designed to test abilities following right-hemisphere damage.	Understanding humor is at a high level. Writing sample asks persons to describe a room in their home, which could be problematic for persons residing in nursing homes.
Minnesota Test for Differential Diagnosis of Aphasia (MTDDA; Schuell, 1973)	Auditory abilities, visual and reading abilities, speech and language, math, writing, numerical relations (e.g., making change, setting clock).	Comprehensive test. Well organized. Does not classify type of aphasia.	Can take a long time to administer in its entirety (1.5 to 2.5 hours).

(continues)

Tests for Adults (Continued)

Test	Evaluates	Pros	Cons
Porch Index of Communicative Ability (PICA; Porch, 2001)	Auditory, reading, verbal, gestural, and written abilities.	Comprehensive. Can be given to persons with a variety of neurogenic disorders. Uses a multidimensional scoring system.	Can take a long time to administer. Extensive training (40 hours) in order to accurately administer and score test.
Reading Comprehension Battery for Aphasia, 2nd edition (RCBA-2; LaPointe & Horner, 1998)	Single-word comprehension, reading short phrases and answering questions, synonyms, sentence comprehension, paragraph comprehension, factual and inferential comprehension, morphosyntactic reading, letter discrimination, letter naming, letter recognition.	Is generally straightforward to administer. Testing materials for clients are in large, bold print. Can be administered in approximately 30 minutes.	Limited normative data available. Supplemental tests can be confusing to administer.
Revised Token Test (RTT; McNeil & Prescott, 1978)	Auditory processing inefficiencies associated with brain damage, aphasia, and language/learning disabilities.	Materials are included. Is sensitive to impairments that may not be evident during observation. Can detect mild auditory comprehension impairments that other standardized tests cannot.	Administering and scoring may be confusing initially. Can take a long time to administer and score.

Instrument	Areas Assessed	Features	Considerations
RIC Evaluation of Communication Problems in Right-Hemisphere Dysfunction–Revised (RICE-R; Halper, Cherney, Burns, & Mogil, 1996)	Characteristics of pragmatics (nonverbal and verbal) including intonation, facial expression, eye contact, gestures, conversation initiation, turn-taking, topic maintenance, and response length.	Developed specifically to assess cognitive communicative problems in persons with right-hemisphere damage. Provides structure to informal observations. Allows clinicians to consider individual differences and compare current performance with premorbid characteristics.	Training is necessary to increase reliable use of the included rating scale.
Rivermead Behavioral Memory Test, 3rd edition (RBMT-III; Wilson et al., 2008)	Orientation, story recall, face and picture recognition, remembering appointments, names, and a message to deliver.	Can be administered in approximately 30 minutes. Includes immediate and delayed recall.	Tasks may not adequately measure the various memory problems that patients may encounter in everyday situations.
Ross Information Processing Assessment, 2nd edition (RIPA-2; Ross-Swain, 1996)	Immediate and recent memory, long-term memory, orientation, reasoning and problem-solving abilities.	Assesses many different cognitive linguistic areas. Directions are easy to follow for clinicians and clients.	Patients may not be as familiar with some of the figurative language included or historical questions asked (e.g., don't cry over spilled milk, who was Helen Keller).
Ross Information Processing Assessment–Geriatric (RIPA-G; Ross-Swain & Fogle, 1996)	Immediate and recent memory, remote memory, spatial orientation, reasoning, orientation, problem solving, activities for independence (e.g., questions asking what one would do if in the bathroom and needed help or if call light was not working).	Designed specifically for adults aged 65 and older. Assesses many different cognitive linguistic areas.	Persons receiving home-based services may have difficulty answering questions that pertain to being at a hospital or healthcare facility.

(continues)

Tests for Adults (*Continued*)

Test	Evaluates	Pros	Cons
Scales of Cognitive Ability for Traumatic Brain Injury (SCATBI; Adamovich & Henderson, 1992)	Orientation, organization, perception/discrimination, recall, and reasoning.	Standardized on a sample of persons with head injuries and a group of adults with no history of head injury. Includes items for high-functioning persons.	Can take up to 2 hours to administer.
Test of Oral Structures and Functions (TOSF; Vitali, 1986)	Articulation, rate, fluency, voice, nonverbal oral functions, orofacial structures.	Can be used as a screening or as thorough diagnostic tool.	Some tasks may be unfamiliar to the patients.
Western Aphasia Battery–Revised (WAB-R; Kertesz, 2006)	Verbal fluency, auditory comprehension, repetition, naming, reading, writing, apraxia, visuospatial, and calculation abilities.	Includes full battery and bed-side screening. Two different forms. Identifies and classifies aphasia types.	May not consistently classify patients with aphasia. Several materials (20 objects) are not included for test administration.

References

Adamovich, B. B., & Henderson, J. (1992). *Scales of cognitive ability for traumatic brain injury.* East Moline, IL: LinguiSystems.

Bayles, K. A. & Tomoeda, C. K. (1993). *Arizona battery for communication disorders of dementia.* Austin, TX: Pro-Ed.

Dabul, B. (2003). *Apraxia battery for adults* (2nd ed.). Austin, TX: Pro-Ed.

Dworkin, J. P., & Culatta, R. (1980). *Dworkin-culatta oral mechanism examination and treatment System.* Nicholasville, KY: Edgewood Press.

Goodglass, H., Kaplan, E., & Barresi, B. (2001). *Boston diagnostic aphasia examination* (3rd ed.). Philadelphia: Lippincott Williams & Wilkins.

Halper, A. S., Cherney, L. R., Burns, M. S., & Mogil, S. I. (1996). *RIC evaluation of communication problems in right hemisphere dysfunction—revised.* Gaithersburg, MD: Aspen Publication, Inc.

Helm-Estabrooks, N. (1992). *Aphasia diagnostic profiles.* New York: Riverside Publishing Co.

Helm-Estabrooks, N. (2001). *Cognitive linguistic quick test.* San Antonio, TX: The Psychological Corporation.

Helm-Estabrooks, N., Ramsberger, G., Morgan, A. R., & Nicholas, M. (1989). *Boston assessment of severe aphasia.* San Antonio, TX: Special Press, Inc.

Holland, A. L., Frattali, C., & Fromm, D. (1999). *Communication activities of daily Living* (2nd ed.). Austin, TX: Pro-Ed.

Kaplan, E., Goodglass, H., & Weintraub, S. (2001). *Boston naming test* (2nd ed.). Philadelphia: Lippincott Williams & Wilkins.

Keenan, J. S., & Brassell, E. G. (1975). *Aphasia language performance scales.* Murfreesboro, TN: Pinnacle Press.

Kertesz, A. (2006). *The western aphasia battery-revised.* San Antonio, TX: Pearson.

Kleiman, L. J. (2003). *Functional communication profile-revised.* East Moline, IL: LinguiSystems.

LaPointe, L. L., & Horner, J. (1998). *Reading comprehension battery for aphasia.* Austin, TX: Pro-Ed.

Loeb, P. A. (1996). *Independent living scales.* san Antonio, TX: The Psychological Corporation.

Mann, G. (2002). *MASA: The mann assessment of swallowing ability.* Clifton Park, NY: Thomson Delmar Learning.

McNeil, M., & Prescott, T. (1978). *Revised token test.* Austin, TX: Pro-Ed.

Munoz-Sandoval, A. F., Cummins, J., Alvarado, C. G., & Ruef, M. L. (2005). *Bilingual verbal ability tests.* Itasca, IL: Riverside Publishing.

Pimental, P., & Kingsbury, N. A. (2000). *Mini inventory of right brain injury* (2nd ed.). Austin, TX: Pro-Ed.

Porch, B. E. (2001). *Porch index of communicative ability.* Albuquerque, NM: PICA Programs.

Ross-Swain, D. (1996). *Ross information processing assessment* (2nd ed.). Austin, TX: Pro-Ed.

Ross-Swain, D., & Fogle, P. T. (1996). *Ross information processing assessment—geriatric.* Austin, TX: Pro-Ed.

Schuell, H. (1973). *Minnesota test for differential diagnosis of aphasia.* Minneapolis: Lund Press.

Vitali, G. J. (1986). *Test of oral structures and functions.* East Aurora, NY: Slossan Educational Publications.

Wilson, B. A., Greenfield, E., Clare, L., Baddeley, A., Cockburn, J., Watson, P., et al. (2008). *Rivermead behavioral memory test* (3rd ed.). London: Pearson.

Yorkston, K. M., & Beukelman, D. R. (1984). *Assessment of intelligibility of dysarthric speech.* Tigard, OR: C. C. Publications.

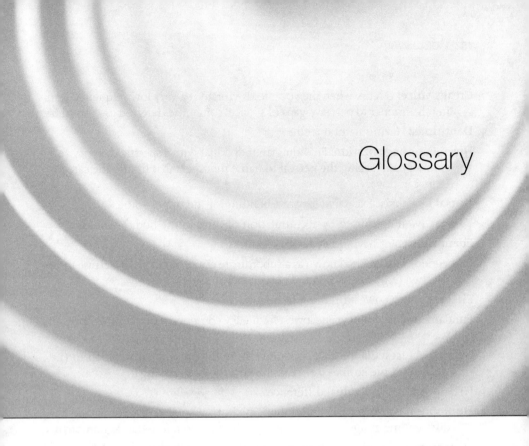

Glossary

Ambiguous referencing: When a pronoun could refer to two possible antecedents (e.g., Harold told his father that *he* has therapy tomorrow).

Anticholinergics: A class of medications that blocks the binding of the neurotransmitter acetylcholine to its receptors in nerve cells. Used to treat a variety of disorders such as gastrointestinal problems (e.g., irritable bowel syndrome), urinary incontinence, and asthma.

Aperiodicity: Irregularity of successive vocal fold vibratory cycles.

Atherosclerotic: A hardening of the arteries caused by the buildup of fatty deposits within the blood vessels, resulting in restricted blood flow.

Atrophy: Muscle that is wasting away or decreasing in size.

Cervical auscultation: Placing a stethoscope along various areas of the neck while a patient swallows; can be useful in determining if an individual aspirates by detecting bubbling sounds during or immediately after swallowing.

Comorbidities: Two or more coexisting diseases or disorders.

Confrontational naming: Showing an individual a series of objects or pictures and asking the person to name the items.

Creaky voice: Occurs when the vocal folds vibrate at a very low frequency, leading the listener to perceive gaps of silence; sometimes referred to as vocal fry.

Dentulous: Having natural teeth.

Divergent categorization: Providing an individual with a specific category (e.g., animals) and asking the person to name members that fit into the category (e.g., cat, dog).

Dorsal kyphosis: Excessive forward bending of the upper spine.

Edema: Swelling caused by accumulation of fluid in the body's tissues.

Edentulous: Not having any teeth; toothless.

Embedded clauses: Also known as a subordinate clause, which is one clause inside another (e.g., The woman *who sang* is her mother).

First formant: Lowest resonant frequency.

Fundamental frequency: The lowest frequency component of a complex periodic wave.

Gerund clauses: Clauses that contain verbs in the present participle form (i.e., verbs with the suffix –ing) (e.g., I heard the baby crying).

Heterogeneity: Individual differences.

Homophones: Words that sound the same but are spelled differently and have different meanings (e.g., sea/see, here/hear); also referred to as homonyms.

Hypercapnia: Condition of too much carbon dioxide in the blood.

Isometric: Muscle contraction that results from placing pressure against a stationary object.

Jitter: Irregularity in the time of vibration of the vocal folds.

Left-branching clauses: Phrases in which the embedded clause occurs to the left of the main clause (e.g., *The gal who runs a nursery school for our church* is awfully young).

Lumina: Cavity of a tubular organ.

Ototoxicity: Damage to the ear; symptoms can include tinnitus, hearing loss, and vertigo.

Paragrammatisms: Speech in which grammatical errors are present, such as the omission of grammatical morphemes.

Paraphasias: Substitution of an incorrect word for the target word.

Parenchyma: Essential or functional elements of an organ.

Patent: Open, clear of obstruction.

Presbycusis: Age-related auditory impairments that often lead to difficulty with speech recognition.

Presbyglutiton: "Old swallow."

Presbylarynges: "Old voice."

Presbyphonia: Age-related degeneration of the voice that is characterized by a bowing of the vocal folds and incomplete glottic closure, leading to a weak, breathy voice.

Propositional density: How much information is conveyed relative to the number of words spoken.

Responsive naming: Individuals are asked to name an item following a short question, usually one related to the function and/or other features of an object (e.g., Question: "What do you write with?" Answer: "Pen").

Right-branching clauses: Phrases in which each clause is produced sequentially and the embedded clause occurs to the right of the main clause (e.g., She's awfully young to be running a nursery for our church).

Sarcopenia: The age-related loss of muscle mass, strength, and function.

Semantic paragraphias: Spelled or written responses that have little resemblance phonologically or visually to the target word, but which are related to the word (e.g., writing "flight" for the word "propeller").

Semantic paraphasias: A word substitution in which the stated word is related to the target word (e.g., person says "fork" when shown a spoon or says "pencil" when shown a pen).

Senescent voice: Aged voice.

Shimmer: Irregularity in the amplitude of vibration of the vocal folds.

Sine qua non: Essential; prerequisite.

Sjögren's syndrome: An autoimmune disease in which there is destruction of the lacrimal and salivary glands, producing dry mouth and dry eyes. Symptoms can include fatigue, joint pain, and depression.

Verbosity: Speech that contains more words than necessary.

Vertebral articulations: Joints that are formed when adjacent vertebrae are connected by ligaments.

Xerostomia: Dry mouth.

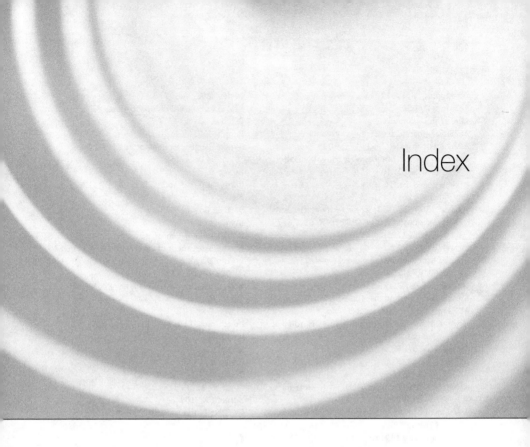

Index